DREAMTELLING, RELATIONS, AND LARGE GROUPS

Robi Friedman is an experienced group analyst and clinician specializing in conflict resolution, and in this important collection of his work, he presents his most innovative concepts.

Dreamtelling is an original approach to the sharing of dreams with partners or within families, exploring how the dreamer's unconscious messages can be communicated, and helping to contain emotional difficulties. The book also explains Friedman's concept relation disorders, which locates dysfunctional behavioural patterns not within intrapsychic issues, but rather as a function of dynamics in group relations. And finally, the book presents the soldier's matrix, a method for conceptualizing processes in highly stressed organizations and societies which are either under existential threat or pursuing glory. In the process of becoming a soldier's matrix, subgroups and nations progressively lose shame, guilt and empathy towards perceived enemies and the Other, and every society member embraces a selfless role. Applying this method to training in groups provides an optimal way out of organizational and national crisis.

The book will be of great interest to group analysts. It will also appeal to psychoanalysts, psychotherapists and clinical psychologists with an interest in conflict resolution.

Robi Friedman, Clinical Psychologist and Group Analyst, was born in Montevideo, Uruguay, and emigrated to Israel at the age of thirteen. He has a private practice in Haifa, Israel; was the co-founder of and teacher at the Israel Institute for Group Analysis; and is the past president of the International Group Analytic Society.

The New International Library of Group Analysis

Series Editor: Earl Hopper

Drawing on the seminal ideas of British, European and American group analysts, psychoanalysts, social psychologists and social scientists, the books in this series focus on the study of small and large groups, organisations and other social systems, and on the study of the transpersonal and transgenerational sociality of human nature. NILGA books will be required reading for the members of professional organisations in the field of group analysis, psychoanalysis, and related social sciences. They will be indispensable for the "formation" of students of psychotherapy, whether they are mainly interested in clinical work with patients or in consultancy to teams and organisational clients within the private and public sectors.

Recent titles in the series

Fairy Tales and the Social Unconscious
The Hidden Language, 1st Edition
Ravit Raufman and Haim Weinberg

Group Analysis in the Land of Milk and Honey
Robi Friedman and Yael Doron

The Linked Self in Psychoanalysis
The Pioneering Work of Enrique Pichon Riviere, 1st Edition
Roberto Losso, Lea S. de Setton and David E. Scharff

On Group Analysis and Beyond
Group Analysis as Meta-Theory, Clinical Social Practice, and Art, 1st Edition
Anastassios Koukis

Dreamtelling, Relations, and Large Groups
New Developments in Group Analysis
Robi Friedman

For further information about this series please visit www.routledge.com/The-New-International-Library-of-Group-Analysis/book-series/KARNNILGA

DREAMTELLING, RELATIONS, AND LARGE GROUPS

New Developments in Group Analysis

Robi Friedman

Routledge
Taylor & Francis Group
LONDON AND NEW YORK

First published 2019
by Routledge
2 Park Square, Milton Park, Abingdon, Oxon OX14 4RN

and by Routledge
52 Vanderbilt Avenue, New York, NY 10017

Routledge is an imprint of the Taylor & Francis Group, an informa business

British Library Cataloguing-in-Publication Data
A catalogue record for this book is available from the British Library

Library of Congress Cataloging-in-Publication Data
A catalog record for this book has been requested

ISBN: 978-1-138-34627-7 (hbk)
ISBN: 978-1-138-34628-4 (pbk)
ISBN: 978-0-429-06041-0 (ebk)

Typeset in Bembo
by Apex CoVantage, LLC

CONTENTS

FOREWORD

Dr Robi Friedman is a clinical psychologist, a psychodynamic psychotherapist who works with persons, couples and families and a group analyst who conducts small clinical groups. He also convenes larger groups in conferences and workshops, as well as in other settings, mainly in the service of conflict resolution, and has developed what he calls the sandwich model, in which a team of group analysts use small and large groups in order to elaborate a particular theme. Dr Friedman was one of the first of us to realize the many implications of the fact that from its inception group analysis, with its roots in European psychoanalysis, in the British study of group dynamics and in the social sciences, was 'relational' in both its theoretical axioms and in its clinical techniques.

The topics of this selection of Friedman's previously published articles range from what he calls dreamtelling, the primacy of interpersonal and transpersonal relations, and the exploration of large groups, to his effort to go beyond what he calls a soldier's matrix, comprised of many of the unconscious restraints and constraints of the socio-cultural-political arrangements of modern Israel. This selection is also a record of his intellectual and professional journey from a position of discontent with the individual and drive-centered paradigms of classical psychoanalysis to a position of creative engagement with the theory of the tripartite matrix as a cornerstone of group analysis. He has become increasingly at home in group analysis as a clinical discipline and as a general field of enquiry.

Born in 1948 in Uruguay to Jewish refugees from Europe during World War II and having experienced racial prejudice from the children and families of Nazi refugees from Germany, Robi emigrated on his own to Israel at 13 years of age. He was joined by his family a year later. At 15 years of age he began his career as an athlete in volleyball, and in 1991 he became the coach of the Israeli National Volleyball Team. He once told me that it was in this context that he learned from experience that it was more important to be a champion than it was to be a star. From 1966 onwards, he served in the Israeli Defense Force, seeing combat in the Six-Day War, the War of Attrition, the Yom Kippur War and the first Lebanese War.

Having studied, trained and worked in Israel and in Zurich, Robi teaches at Haifa University and the Israeli Institute of Group Analysis, of which he was a co-founder. The past president of the Group Analytic Society International and the past president of the Israeli Association of Group Therapy, he is also a senior group analyst at SGAZ, the Zurich Institute of Group Analysis, and supervises group analysis in Israel, Denmark, Germany, Italy, Russia and China. In the context of the International Dialogue Initiative, he co-leads with Dr Vamik Volkan and Lord Alderdice the 'West/Islam dialogues', and has worked in Turkey, Northern Ireland, Ukraine and Russia. I would like to add to this list of accomplishments that Robi is married, a father of three children, and a grandfather of seven.

It is only in retrospect that what in the Old Testament was called a 'sojourn' can be seen to have been a journey, and that the end of a journey can be foretold in its beginning. Similarly, only in retrospect can it be seen that Robi's insight that the essence of dreams is not only in the act of dreaming them, but also in telling them within a particular configuration of relations, involved not only a theoretical and clinical shift, but also a change in his professional and personal identities. Dreamtelling transforms the crucible of a dream from a human body to a communication within a dyad of persons, a family, a community and even within a society as a whole. This new perspective allows the appreciation of the dreamer's relational hope that other people will hear his plea to be recognized and understood, to help keep alive his sense of desirous expectation and to join him in his effort to exercise the transcendent imagination. Robi's study of dreamtelling has evolved into carefully structured workshops which focus on telling dreams in groups and on trying to understand flesh-and-blood dreamers who are attempting to communicate with one another through the medium of their co-created dreams. Of crucial importance is the clinically astute management of the dynamic matrices of the groups in which this activity takes place.

I have been impressed by Robi's conceptualization of the symptoms of personal psychic distress as disorders of relations. A myriad of anxieties is manifest in styles of thinking, feeling and relating to other people in ways that provoke them to respond in complementary, reciprocal and disrupting ways. These responses tend to amplify and magnify the initial symptoms, which have been formed within a relational field in the first place. However, the knowledge and appreciation of the power of the patterns that characterize such vicious circles suggest strategies for clinical interventions and therapeutic modes of relating.

This understanding of dreamtelling and of relational disorders has developed into the study of what Robi calls the soldier's matrix and into his attempts to go beyond it. Of course, a soldier's life is very hard, but a soldier's life is a source of glory as well as traumatic pain, both for the soldier himself and for those he loves and with whom he is involved and interdependent, and vice versa. This is particularly true in a society which must continue to mobilize an army of citizens, and which cannot become dependent on an army of professional soldiers. In a society engaged in chronic war, even birth and death acquire enhanced dramatic meanings, which is a kind of irony – if not a paradox. Holding and containing and being held and contained become continuing preoccupations, and the relations between men and women are infused by the pressures for actual survival.

This book will be invaluable and even inspirational to all group analysts, both students and senior practitioners alike. It conveys a sense of the fecundity of group analysis, especially in its many applications. Dr Robi Friedman has shown us that his own soldier's mufti is a version of Joseph's coat of many colours. In this book he has given us an opportunity to share a collective transitional object.

Earl Hopper, PhD
Series Editor

GENERAL INTRODUCTION

This book presents my published thinking while working in group and individual therapy for almost half a century. My reflections usually arise from using introspection – in the same way that we investigate the dynamics and contents of our interactions with patients. When I arrive at insights about my clinical work, I then try to relate them to theories that I know. But my main guide has been my own experience and emotional compass; it has influenced me more than any theoretical approach. I think this may be the reason why my perspective on dreaming, psychopathology in disordered relations and my views on societies under stress are considered creative, perhaps 'different', and have a personal touch.

My own personal background is part and parcel of this 'thinking process'. I live in a country at war. I have experienced numerous wars and the existential tension in Israel. Together with my combat experience, it seems to have facilitated an investigation and reflection on the complicated emotional situations involved in societies under stress – invoked by trauma or the promise of glory. The soldier's matrix is a social construct, as I will describe below, where unified thinking and a restriction on reflection promote the increasingly blind pursuit of leaders and slogans. For me personally, it was a challenge to admit that societies at war or under stress always involve fundamental feelings of glory. This taboo must be named as a central social as well as personal motivation.

I grew up in my mother's Jewish-German family, who had to live through the painful transition of feeling like the Fatherland's heroes, to later being accused of treason. This allowed me to understand the present German anti–soldier's matrix. I believe that having been exposed to my family's painful processes and the efforts to overcome them also helped me, later in life, to distance myself from my early total identifications. I feel fortunate to have achieved this distance – I believe it helped me to a greater extent than through my contribution to the conceptualization of social aspects of the soldier's matrix. In addition, the years I worked and studied in Zurich also contributed to my ability to enter and exit my social matrix. While writing my PhD (Friedman, 1977), which helped me to understand how important Jewish socialization was for the horrible traumas of the Holocaust, I had ample space to struggle with my Jewish and Israeli identity.

Growing up just after the end of the Second World War, in a family of immigrants, I observed them in the process of adapting to a new country and to a difficult language. To add to this, most of them also had their hands full with overcoming their Holocaust experiences, which made it possible for me to meet post-trauma and pathology from very early on. Without words, I knew of their suffering and hopes and that their craziness was to a large extent man-made. Their traumas influenced every piece of interaction and every inch of how they developed in new relationships. It certainly helped me to understand how close people share and distribute pathology. Thus, when I finally could conceptualize relation disorders, following S.H. Foulkes's (1990) ideas about the 'location' of pathology, it was for me an 'unthought known' (Bollas, 1987), an unconscious and unspoken truth which rang a bell in me, as the audience and witness of a familiar nightmare.

My approach to dreams has certainly been influenced by having always been personally close to my dreams. I feel lucky that my dreaming is so often available to me, and even luckier to be able to share some dreams with partners because I felt it was always helpful in my development. Dreamtelling is not an 'invention' – but rather an application of my human and social instincts. Freud's relationship with Fliess (Masson, 1986), in which he shared his dreams and later his book *The Interpretation of Dreams*, seems to me a natural result of these relations. I define dreamtelling as the whole process of elaborating excessively strong emotions through first 'dreaming' them, while trying to 'digest' them internally, then waking up, remembering the dream and later, through finding a partner with whom to share and hopefully discuss the dream.

Dreamtelling fascinates on at least three levels: all of them may be called relational. It is fascinating when we, dreamers and 'dreamers who dream the dream' (Grotstein, 1979), find together a meaning beneath the manifest content. It is also fascinating when a dream rings a faint bell, and when this murmur transforms into music for all involved. Then, a 'moment of meeting' occurs, and a very intimate human encounter has taken place. And I add the communicative fascination as the third way in which hidden demands for influence on the relations and requests for containment create a communicating environment. Dreamtelling expands the limits of what we know about human communication and relations.

Fortunately, more than a few colleagues and friends have responded to my way of approaching dreams with support and understanding. Some of these friends, like Claudio Neri and Malcolm Pines, have even helped me to translate my work into words that explain my thoughts and touch some hearts. My Freudian background forced me to overcome the wish to keep an individual monopoly on dreams. My own approach may be considered as complementing the 'private' classical approach. From the very conception of my ideas on dreams, their value lay in the relations. Even if Bion did not work with dreams in groups – and Donald Meltzer (1983), who supervised some of my work, would turn in his grave if he knew that we would elaborate dreams, but not in the protected dyadic space – I think Bion often approached dreams similarly. It was especially Morgenthaler's (1986) thinking which supported my conceptualization of my own contribution to working on dreams that I soon called dreamtelling. It was in classes at Rome's La Sapienza University that my work with dreams in relations was first called: 'Friedman dreamtelling'. I felt my approach was accepted and supported, which helped me to further elaborate it. Today I think that dreams are usually conceived in relations and then shortly worked through alone, in a first 'dreaming' step. Later, in a second step, if possible, dreams are shared in relations, for communicative and 'digestive' reasons. Dreamtelling can make a whole group pregnant, as it often starts an exchange of elaboration, where resonance to another's latent and manifest dream material creates a space in which the unconscious is touched upon.

I know that it takes a while to accept that dreams are so intimately connected with relations. We dream about someone, with someone and may share it and elaborate it through someone. Our container, our digestive apparatus, is not only inside, but also outside. That is what makes relations so interesting. Such relations may become even more interesting when they create further dreaming. Where there is a container there will be dreams.

Using introspection to investigate the quality of our relations often proves painful, because we too easily detect how dysfunctional patterns of behaviour are influenced by human relations. My view of pathology and health was significantly formed by two unique group cultures: sport and the army. One of the most salient qualities in professional sport and in the army is that women and men constantly change groups and thereby have to adapt to different relations and settings. Often, in the most important games I played in my life, the final and optimal team combination was not the one which started. In the army, especially in difficult situations, soldiers and commanders will survive if they adapt to rapidly changing teams. This makes it possible to observe scapegoats in one team achieve a significantly better positioning in another group and vice versa: kings who prove so inefficient that they become scapegoats on the verge of rejection. Time and again I observed how relations in pairs and groups affect sanity and create dysfunctional behaviour patterns. Individual pathology does not explain satisfactorily our clinical experience of pathology. With time I also understood Foulkes's hypothesis that viewing pathology as relations-made is frightening and guilt provoking.

As Foulkes had not gone deeper into this issue, probably because he himself avoided the struggles and opposition, which I came to experience later, it became important to me to try to adumbrate categories of relation disorders. I used my interpretation of Agazarian's (1994) conceptualization, following her research on the developmental journey that groups take. Research on groups found that they develop some autonomy after feeling dependent, and security after feeling very anxious in the beginning. Trust in others and a healthy interdependency is also a main development. I used her research to characterize each of the four relation disorders by the ill-containment of central social emotions. These emotional social situations were dependency, aggression and rejection, identification and positioning in the group's centre or margins. All relation disorders describe reciprocal and chronic relations between the group's centre and its subgroups, which also means that the therapeutic approach is relational too – one always has to approach the two sides of a disorder and their relationship.

In the last section of the book I present some of my thoughts about the already mentioned soldier's matrix. This is a special social structure of a society under stress from existential threats and hopes for glory. The concept points to the recruitment of all members of society in a huge effort in which there is massification of thought, selfless sacrifice and over-identification with the aims of an organization or society. Those living in it progressively lose emotional abilities like feelings of guilt, shame and empathy. The concept of the soldier's matrix summarizes social and personal processes which I understood while working with individuals and groups in Germany and Israel. Germany impressed me by having implemented such tremendous changes after literally drowning during the Second World War in the worst ever soldier's matrix. After being, time and again, influenced by the trauma and glory of war gods over hundreds of years, German children and grandchildren of the war generation achieved a separation process from their soldier's matrix, probably during a phase which I call the 'anti–soldier's matrix'.

Israel, on the other hand, seems to find itself in rather extreme adherence to the soldier's matrix. During the last half century, far from progressively enjoying a more secure and pleasant environment, Israel's growing economic and military strength is not necessarily felt as a relief, but as a necessary asset in order to continue surviving. The soldier's matrix is a Moloch, continuously demanding more selfless sacrifice, which rather restricts its members, increasingly, devouring their liberties of deed and thought, marginalizing and rejecting some of its own citizens.

I will try to describe this society and tentatively propose the sandwich model, a tool which mixes the small and large group in order to cope with the difficulties of reflecting on one's own culture. The sandwich model makes it possible to reflect and maybe overcome over-identification with the soldiers' matrix, estrangement, splits and other social maladies. The participation in a large group may facilitate a developmental process in which members have more choice and liberty to move closer and away from one's own matrix.

One of the main points which pervades this book is the unique contribution of groups to therapy. I believe, for example, that optimal indications for therapy have to take group therapy into account. I also learned from my experience as an individual and group therapist that very often, pathology can be best cured in the environment it was engendered. Disorders caused by social interactions should be optimally treated in groups, after, before or complementary to individual therapy. Optimal treatment must provide a space in which dysfunctional patterns re-emerge and can be treated by insight and practice. The four relation disorders are examples of difficulties which can be best treated inside a group setting.

The understanding that humans are related to one another through a thousand unseen ties and in an unconscious boundary-less way is a thread connecting the whole book. This thread goes through dreaming, dreamtelling and relation disorders – it is all about being influenced in a society, in an intersubjective or what group analysis calls 'transpersonal' way of communicating clinical vignettes, theoretical thoughts and analysis of processes to try to make belonging to a group understandable, both in its development and its difficulties. I also provide personal examples which may help to connect to the roots of my own perspective and positions. Groups may help growth as well as cause destruction. They enable us to achieve aims which are impossible to reach individually. We need more ways to learn how the participants' joint power can be used creatively to promote transformation and growth.

References

Agazarian, I. (1994) The Phases of Group Development and the Systems-centred Group. In M. Pines and V. Schermer (Eds.), *Ring of Fire.* London: Routledge.
Bollas, C. (1987) *The Shadow of the Object.* London: Free Association.
Grotstein, J.S. (1979) Who Is the Dreamer Who Dreams the Dream and Who Is the Dreamer Who Understands It. *Contemporary Psychoanalysis*, 15(1).
Foulkes, S.H. (1990) *Selected Papers: Psychoanalysis and Group Analysis.* Edited by E. Foulkes. London: Karnac.
Friedman, R. (1977) *Das Problem der Aggression und seine psychologische Deutung in der Tradition des judischen Denkens.* Zollikon: Doktorarbeit, Universität Zurich.
Masson, J. (1986) *The Complete Letters of Sigmund Freud to Wilhelm Fliess, 1887–1904.* Harvard: Belknap Press.
Meltzer, D. (1983) *Dream-Life.* Perthshire, Scotland: Clunie Press.
Morgenthaler, F. (1986) *Der Traum.* Frankfurt: Qumran.

PART I

Dreams and dreamers in relation and some research on dreamtelling in families

INTRODUCTION TO PART I

Introduction

Dreamtelling

It all started with my connection to my dreaming and my interest in the relations between the dream's content and the relational context in which it is remembered and told. Two 'events' helped me to define my own thinking on dreamtelling (Friedman, 2008). The first was when my son was about three or four years old, and often woke up from what seemed to be a nightmare. His nocturnal cries made me jump out of my bed and rush into his room. He usually returned to sleep in a moment – while I was left worried, especially if this repeated itself in the same night. I learned from this 'interaction' about the non-verbal communication of anxiety and panic, and even more about the possibility that feelings can be shared between a dreamer and his audience. Later I understood that these are more familiar situations than we think. I called my son's communication a 'request for containment'; I understood that I was the 'container-on-call' and that there was a very deep relation between the two of us.

The other event which helped me to understand the deeper communicative aspects of dreamtelling was a patient's story: he fell for a young woman in a party, but could not find enough courage to approach her directly. Back home, he dreamt about her with red lips, which seemed to be waiting for a kiss . . . and in his dream they did indeed have a passionate kiss. Although first his dream just felt like 'wishful thinking' there was a completely additional side to the dream in this story. In our area, party participants used to meet on the beach the next afternoon. Then, 'armed' with this dream, he found the courage to approach the young woman and conquer her heart by sharing his dream with her. It was only much later that I could conceptualize what seemed to be a banality: the dream's power to demand to influence a relationship. Understanding the 'told' dream's unconscious communication as a wish to change the relations with the audience helped me to further clarify 'transformative' sides in dreamtelling. Dreams are not only informative, but have the power to transform relations. Later I understood the general clinical value of understanding much of human communications as 'requests for containment' and 'demands for transformation of relations'.

By dreamtelling I refer to a whole elaboration process, which starts with a dreamer's autonomous effort to elaborate excessive emotions during sleep, and finishes by further elaborating these excessively strong emotions through sharing the dream with a co-operative audience. Dreams may be remembered and told to others, and also resonate with others. While usually dreams told in therapy seem to request an interpretation, in my clinical experience I found that not every dreamer is ready for an interpretation, nor are the relations with the dreamer ready for touching the unconscious. Finally, we have to acknowledge that simple human resonance is often more needed than deep interpretation (Friedman, 2006).

This insight helped me to define what it means to work 'formatively': when we feel the dreamer is in some danger of fragmentation, or in crisis, etc. We should use the dream told in order to first strengthen the dreamer's Self. Dreamtelling can call for a first 'forming' or structuring of the relation between all participants. That is one reason why I often suggest that our reactions to a dream told should be 're-dreaming the dream' as if it was the listener's own dream.

Dreams are the result of a special kind of mental 'digestion' of excessively threatening and/or exciting emotions. It is an adaptive system, functional and natural for humans like the process of breathing oxygen. Later they may be adapted into our being or thinking – sometimes in order to enjoy them. By magically translating emotions and thoughts into stories, scripts, images, known or wished relations and voices, dreams are created. Research maintains that most probably our unconscious elaboration makes use of our whole lifetime experience, by comparing past and present situations.

My first professional encounter with dreams was influenced by the classical approach to the dream as a text. What first drew my attention were the dream's contents, I suppose much in in the same way as Freud's (1900) traditional, 'diagnostic' approach, which I later renamed as 'informative'. Many of us who are interested in dreams, are first fascinated by unveiling the unconscious, to get more knowledge of the dreamer's psyche, to decipher latent contents like the Rosetta Stone. Soon another interest awoke in me and I asked: In which unique way does the dream itself reveal how the dreamer copes with his difficulties? Together with Morgenthaler (1986) and others, I felt the creation of the dream and its structure would characterize the dreamer more than we thought.

But the information which interested me quickly led me into more interactional realms. Firstly, I asked if every dreamer is able to profit from deep interpretation. My clinical experience showed this is in no way so. In this book I try to give guidance as to who could be harmed from interpretation, and how to determine this ahead of time. Dreamtelling also makes it potentially possible to find partners who could co-operate. Dreams send powerful conscious and unconscious messages which influence the dreamer's relation with the audience. As we discovered in our research, this is also true of new partnerships.

I learned that not all of the dream's contents are told into the transference, and therefore are not exclusively directed at the listening therapist. Although this often happens, dreamtelling is more connected to requests for containment and further elaboration. Dreamtelling is also more than merely a tool for the elaboration of excessive emotions, but the creation of relations and partnerships and their transformation. This alone makes dreamtelling a fascinating and complex interpersonal event. Dreams suddenly went beyond being 'the royal way to the dreamer' and became 'the royal way to the dreamer's psyche through his relations with others'. The strangest part was when it became clear that the dreamer was not only dreaming for himself but had been called upon to elaborate emotional difficulties of others too. It is always his own problem, but this new understanding that our dreaming may 'borrowed' by those close to us is actually mind blowing. A child, a friend or a patient may ask the dreamer to digest his uncontained problem. In therapy groups it makes shared work reciprocally significant.

Working with dreams does not need magical endowment or witchcraft. It can be learned. As a rule, when there is a container, dreams are better remembered and shared. When dreams are shared in families or groups, they overcome modern culture's malady of disconnection with our inner life. Participants in 'dream-groups' seem to get in touch with the dreams' complexity and richness and progressively befriend dreamtelling to develop a better elaboration of difficult emotions. I learned much from dream-groups, where the therapeutic work is done through sharing dreams and responding to them, as if they were 'your own dream'. In therapeutic groups which include dreamtelling, the relations become qualitatively different.

The theatre of the mind (Resnik, 2002) becomes the dream stage where group experiences both influence and are elaborated. S.H. Foulkes (1964) himself did not move far from the traditional early psychoanalytic thinking on dreams which emphasized contents. In fact, dreamtelling works in a way that promotes identification processes with the dreamer, and can be considered to be a model for group-analytic work. It makes optimal use of the group as a source for mirroring and resonance, creating within the group a certain music around dreams, which has to be played and heard to connect to it emotionally.

The chapter on research describes an investigation we made at Haifa University asking 100 men and 100 women about their family history, personal past, and the present patterns of dreamtelling. Particularly interesting were connections made between parental containment of their children's dreams and subsequent ability to relate to the inner world in general and dreams in particular. There was significant evidence of transgenerational transmission of the ability to share dreams. After we understood the developmental significance of sharing dreams, it also became clear that most modern families do not have the know-how to listen and react to children's dreams in a way which furthers communication, rather than shame, guilt or manipulation. Individuals, couples and families who own some ability to work in a dreamtelling 'fashion' seemed to profit from great emotional communicative advantages. For example, men in love tell unusually more dreams to their new partners, something which also shows that they feel to have found a container and are unconsciously prone to influence the growing relationship.

My own long story with conflict resolution started more than 20 years ago with a difficulty to shake the hand of a Palestinian professional. In the years after that, I went through a lot of pain and elaboration of many difficult feelings, especially hate, shame and the most difficult feeling of all: guilt. The 'guilt war': the ability to accuse the other side along with the difficulty to accept one's own guilt (Friedman, 2015). This seems to me to be the most significant obstacle to talks with former 'enemies'. It requires not only personal transformative processes to overcome the destructivity of such a war, but also a special social situation which supports the feelings of guilt. In many settings, I have tried and still do try to meet hate and accusations from the 'other side'. Dreams where more than one side is represented helped me to be able to understand and contain the 'other' side and the feelings aroused. In fact, we can often see how dreams, when elaborated as a dialogue between differing and conflicting aspects in ourselves and in society, become as close to a conflict resolution dialogue as they can be.

References

Foulkes, S.H. (1964) *Therapeutic Group Analysis*. London: Allen and Unwin. Reprinted 1984. London: Karnac.

Freud, S. (1900) *The Interpretation of Dreams* (ch. 6–7. Standard Edition 4–5). London: Hogarth Press.

Friedman, R. (2006) *The Dream Narrative as an Interpersonal Event – Research Results*. funzionegamma. La Sapienza, Univ. of Rome. www.funzionegamma.edu/inglese/currentnumber/friedman.asp

Friedman, R. (2008) Dreamtelling as a Request for Containment – Three Uses of Dreams in Group Therapy. *International Journal of Group Psychotherapy*, 58(3): 327–344.

Friedman, R. (2015) Using the Transpersonal in Dream-telling and Conflicts. *Group Analysis*, 48(1): 1–16.

Morgenthaler, F. (1986) *Der Traum*. Frankfurt: Qumran.

Resnik, S. (2002) Reflections on Dreams. The Implications for Groups. In C. Neri, M. Pines and R. Friedman (Eds.), *Dreams in Group Psychotherapy* (pp. 197–209). London: Jessica Kingsley Publishers.

1

DREAMTELLING AS A REQUEST FOR CONTAINMENT

Three uses of dreams in group therapy[1]

This chapter introduces a clinical theory for working with dreams, hypothesizing three functions of dreams told in the clinical setting: the informative, the formative, and the transformative. Group-analytic and relational theories are employed to focus on two functions of dreamtelling that are both unconscious and intersubjective: the (unconscious) implied requests for containment and for influence on relations with the dream-audience.

Differentiating between dreaming and dreamtelling

Freud (1900) was the first to conceptualize dreams as 'a way of thinking', and many psychoanalytic theorists, including Jung (1974), Bion (1962), Meltzer (1983), Kohut (1984) and Ogden (1996), have followed in his footsteps, considering dreaming as a coping mechanism. There seems to be general theoretical consensus that a dream is dreamed in order to work through emotional difficulties in the dreamer's mind. Dreaming is an intrapsychic process that helps the dreamer cope with mental content that in waking life might be experienced as too threatening or exciting. As such and as Freud (1900) posited, dreams can provide the 'royal road' to knowledge about the dreamer's unconscious. Since Freud, generations of therapists have invested in deciphering the dream's hieroglyphs and secrets hidden beneath its manifest contents, and many consider the revelation of those secrets the closest that we can get to the dreamer's true self. In the context of the therapy group, a dream is also considered the 'royal way' of understanding the latent desires and conflicts of the group as a whole and those of other participants besides the dreamer.

In contrast to dreaming, which is regarded primarily as an intrapsychic and autonomous function, dreamtelling is always an interpersonal event that results from an unconscious choice to share disguised or vague information. Dreamtelling raises the intriguing questions as to whom we tell a dream and why – that is, what is consciously and unconsciously expected and wanted from the other in telling the dream. While only the self is available to contain the dream during dreaming, in dreamtelling the other can help contain the dream. The recipient can elaborate on the dream content to help work through undigested emotions and unprocessed dynamics.

Dreaming may be considered the intrapsychic phase of elaboration of emotional excesses, while dreamtelling may be understood as a complementary interpersonal phase, similarly aiming to further digest the unaccomplished elaboration of emotional tensions first tackled while dreaming. I call this function of dreamtelling a 'Request for Containment' (Friedman, 2000). If the dreaming phase proves unsatisfactory in resolving internal tensions, it may be followed by another – now interpersonal – chance to elaborate something left uncontained in the dream. One condition for this is that the dreamer finds an 'elaborating' partner, receptive of the request and capable of a further containment effort. Dreamtelling's second intersubjective function is to significantly exert (usually unconscious) influence on the relationship with the listener (Friedman, 2004). Dreams told are meant to have a strong impact on the interpersonal processes, as will be illustrated below. Limiting our attention as group therapists only to the contents of the dream and the internal world of the dreamer may be reductive and an oversimplification of the complex interpersonal processes involved in dreamtelling.

The three uses of dreams: informative, formative and transformative

In addition to the differentiation between dreaming and dreamtelling, clinically working with dreams can be understood from three perspectives: the analysis of dreams to assess or diagnose a person or group – the informative use; to strengthen the dreamer's ego or structure of the self, or, analogously, to enhance the working capacities of the group – the formative use; and understanding dreamtelling as a powerful interpersonal communication that changes relationships with the dream's audience – the transformative use. The first, informative perspective is the classic approach to explore and interpret the dream's content and structures to raise consciousness or expand knowledge about the dreamer and his/her internal world. A dream reported in the therapy group can illuminate heretofore unknown depths of the individual and also of the group entity. A second, formative use of the reported dream is to therapeutically strengthen the dreamer's processing capacities, particularly when regression and trauma threaten to fragment the self. This non-interpretative approach is also helpful to deal with the immature developing personality evident in children's dreams. Finally, the third, transformative aspect signifies that dreamtelling may enact wishes to influence a relationship with the audience in a particular way. The therapist needs to attend to all three dimensions and should be aware of the complexity of such an endeavour for all group participants.

Clinical illustration: biking in the therapy group

A participant in a twice-weekly therapy group reports the following dream:

> The whole therapy group is mountain biking on Mount Carmel. I (the dreamteller) ride first, near the group conductor. Then I start to ride faster than everyone, scouting the way and returning many times to the group in order to make sure that everything is OK.

This patient's dreaming may be considered a first step in the containment of excessive threats and excitement (Bion, 1962), in this case, the conflictual excitement and fear of fulfilling his desire for closeness to the leader and beating the other participants by being the best biker. By telling his dream, he acknowledges in the presence of his therapy group both his intrapsychic effort to cope with finding his place in the group and his competing tendencies. This man, an independent professional in his late 30s, has had chronic difficulties establishing authentic, intimate and lasting relationships. He grew up with what he perceived as a 'wonderful', but actually frightening and domineering, mother who very often humiliated both him and his father. As revealed in the therapy, there were two dominant emotional preoccupations: (1) in spite of his own achievements in his professional field, he deeply envied his very successful brother, who seemed to be his mother's favourite, and (2) his sexuality, manifested primarily by extensive masturbatory activities or superficial relationships with women. He and the six other patients, all in their 30s, had been participating in a twice-a-week therapeutic group for three years. His efforts to feel included in the group, which had usually been repulsed by a very critical subgroup who felt that his behaviour was disingenuous and inhibited, experienced a turning point after the dreamtelling, a disclosure that was considered to be more open and honest. Until then they had pitied him for being a bright but immature young man who had to pose and put on (clothes, words) to cover for his lonely, perverted and emotionally superficial role in life.

His dream indirectly informs the audience of his internal dynamics and conflicts. He demands to be first, has difficulty in relying on others, especially the leader, but at the same time suffers from separation from others. We assume that the intrapsychic process while dreaming in which the dreamer tried to cope with the conflict between his competition with me as group leader and his needs for a secure bond was to no avail. Because he had been unsuccessful on his own, I proposed the idea that he bring the dream to the group as an implicit request for the containment of his conflict.

I have described elsewhere how dreamtelling may also have an impact on the future relationship of the dreamer with the dream-audience (Friedman, 2004). By telling the dream, the dreamer not only signifies his relationship with the group, which feels to him to be marginal in contrast to his wished-for intimacy with me as the leader, but also immediately influences it through the implicit ambivalent message. He seems to create a split relationship with the 'less-important' group on the one hand and with me, the conductor, for him the only significant person in the group. This complex competition and separation dynamic is conveyed through his back-and-forth motions to the group and me.

As the group discussion following his account of his dream progressed, the dreamer's ambivalent interest for both closeness and rejection led the group to distance themselves, leaving him alone in his struggle. Being insensitive to his exclusion of the group, while asking for closeness to me, he was responded to essentially with a cold shoulder and devaluing reaction. To his effort to explain his biking to and fro, a woman reacted dismissively by saying, 'Words, words, words . . .' and another man, who also bikes, boasted about his own biking accomplishments. Now the essence of the dream seemed to be totally enacted in the group: the patient's solitude and distance from the group together with his ambivalence toward me were not only reflected in the dream's contents but also evident in the group process. As this process unfolded, the group attacked the dreamer for his 'arrogance' and what they felt to be his detached and pushy competitive behaviour together with his immature dependence on the group conductor.

On psychic permeability, dreaming for others and 'being together' in a group

In the psychoanalytic literature, dreaming has been considered as an exclusively intrapsychic process. However, dreaming as a process that represents containment and elaboration of difficulties may be more than a purely individual activity. Through psychic permeability and identificatory tendencies, the individual dreamer uses others' containment and elaborative abilities to help digest difficulties. We do not dream exclusively our own conflicts but also others' problems – dreams can be dreamed 'for' other people. Difficulties of close ones may touch, move and activate a related and identifying dreamer. A mother may consciously and unconsciously tackle her child's problems by dreaming about them and the same may be said of other significant relationships – through identifications, the therapist may dream something for his/her patient and vice versa. A difficulty may be dreamed by someone in group therapy or a family, because he/she has a greater ability to work through it than his/her troubled partner(s). The dreamer's identification with the material and his greater capability to dream a difficulty for the other combine with presupposed closeness, based on psychic permeability and intersubjective communication, in order to launch the elaboration process during dreaming. Group interaction encompasses a whole range of surface to deep interpersonal, intersubjective interactions, from presenting and witnessing difficult emotions to elaborating and associating to them, and to influencing each other in more ways than consciousness permits us to know. This communicative and elaborative interchange mediated by projections and identifications is defined as the 'container-contained' process (Bion, 1962; Ogden, 1979; Rafaelsen, 1996).

In our clinical example, it could be said that this patient's dream is used by others in the group in order to work through a certain interpersonal dynamic, especially concerns over who the leader's favourite is in the group. What is posited here is the idea that the dream told in the group may be voicing and elaborating an issue affecting not only the dreamer but those in his social environment. As such, it offers the chance for a deeper dialogue in the group if there is an openness to share and engage in an 'elaborating partnership' (Friedman, 2002a) through the dream.

I am suggesting that the patient had dreamed the question, 'Who is close to the group conductor?' but was unable to resolve the tension stemming from this concern by himself. The disguises of the manifest dream and the latent significance of symbols such as riding a bicycle, scouting and displacements pictured in the dream's content shed light on the dreamer as well as the group's moods and motivations. This dreamer, because of his unique personality and relationship patterns, had the ability to identify with these problems and had become a (partial) container of these emotional difficulties, dreaming them both for himself and for others in the group. Conceptualizing the dreamtelling in this way helps to understand the resonance of listeners to particular dreams, and why the group so easily relates to a personal dream, which, taken up as the dominant subject for discourse, represents something significant in others' psychic lives.

Where there is a container, there are dreams. If there is hope for personal growth in a constructive relationship, a dream may be told in an effort to complete an unsuccessful elaboration during dreaming. The dream is not told or shared with others if there is an anticipation of rejection by the listener.

The classic approach: the informative use of dreams

Dreams serve therapists, friends and family members as a reservoir of information, understanding and deep knowledge about the dreamer and his relationship with them. These elements are usually retrieved from the dream's contents but we can additionally use the dream's structure, thinking about not only what is said but how it is said. While the Freudian approach to dream interpretation tries to detect dynamics and conflicts disguised in the dream's content, other 'informative' aspects have been developed. For example, object relations theory offers the view that split-off, unaccepted feelings are represented in the 'not-me' dream contents. According to this formulation, the dream is essentially an effort to ease the grip of unbearable feelings, mainly through the projection of these threatening parts of the self ('me') in(to) external objects ('not me'). Dreamers may be haunted by aggressors, threatened by envious others, or persecuted by sexual temptations. This process of dis-covering hidden meanings in our nightly pictures and texts in order to 're-own' them seems to have remained the prevailing psychoanalytical approach. Remarkably, the general approach to working with dreams in group therapy is very similar to this individual approach. Even those contributions that approach the dreams told as 'group dreams' usually treat them in a fairly classic informative style – that is, helping to illuminate the internal world of the dreamer. However, because the manifest content of the dream contains elements of the group cannot by itself define a 'group dream', – it seems more important to help participants relate to dreamed material, thus promoting it to the 'dream of the group'. 'Dreaming the dream' (Grotstein, 1979) together gives a unique advantage to group therapy because of the multifocal responses, and facilitating this capacity has to be the ultimate objective of the group therapist. Whether called feedback or resonance, sharing the 'striking a cord' to the other and his/her unconscious is a unique reciprocal tool available in groups.

Additional parameters to the usual informative aspects can be found in the analysis and interpretation of the dream's structure, which reflects the abilities and structure of the dreamer's ego (Friedman, 2002b). The organization of the dream's narrative, its script and story, including the number and nature of its characters, may give us clues about the dreamer's personality and internalized interpersonal patterns, which may be enacted in the group. Investigating the roles of the dream's protagonists may contribute to both a deeper knowledge of the dreamer's internalized group and his/her coping patterns with conflictual relations. The dream's protagonists are 'recruited' because of their ability to contain exciting or threatening emotions, thus functioning as 'containing roles' (Agazarian, 1994). They are objects 'used' by the dreamer[2] for working-through purposes by a process that I have called projective-identification-in-the-dream (Friedman, 2002b; Ogden, 1979; Rafaelsen, 1996).

I have previously called the informative approach 'diagnostic' in order to stress that the classic use of the material retrieved from a dream was to establish the dreamer's psychodiagnosis and facilitate self-knowledge (Friedman, 2002b). Similar diagnostic uses of dreams may be found in object relations theory (Grotstein, 2002; Bion, 1992) or in self-psychology (Stone and Karterud, 2006), as well as other psychoanalytic schools. In this latter approach the dreamer's ego ability to achieve coherence in his/her self-state dreams is examined; dream contents are investigated for relationships having self-object functions.

Looking at our dream vignette from an informative/diagnostic perspective, the dreamer's representation of me as the group leader, as elaborated in the group, is as someone who is able to tolerate both aggressively tinged competition and the patient's ambivalent distancing and approaching. It is as if our dreamer, who grew up with a very dominating and frightening mother and brother and a devalued and insignificant father, informs us in the dream about the fresh interpersonal experience that he tries to achieve through the group. It is also important to evaluate the dream's organizational quality: a narrative that includes organized movement (energy) and unambiguous characters that seem sufficiently engaged with each other are usually signs of a strong-enough ego, which makes disclosing and depth work possible. The higher the level of structure in the dream, the more safety is felt in the group to engage in a free discourse on the dream's personal and interpersonal significance.

The manner and context of dreamtelling provide additional clues about the dreamer and his/her social relations. In the present vignette, the dream was told in an open and forthright manner that offered ample space for a dialogue to further understanding of important relationship patterns and transference phenomena within the group. For example, some sessions after the dream report, I responded to a participant's anger towards the dreamer's insensitivity in the group, that his biking dream has some similarity with the biblical dream told by Joseph to his brothers. His brothers became so infuriated that they threw him into a pit and sold him into slavery. Two sessions later, a woman in the group commented that my reference to Joseph's dream helped her to understand her feelings toward our dreamer. She shared her own fear as well as her wish to feel close to me. Clearly, themes of envy, competition and conflicts about closeness were evoked by the dream and its telling in the group.

There is much to learn from the context in which a dream is told. Consider, for example, the difference between a written dream told by a patient at the beginning of a session and one offered in the last few minutes. A reported dream is a communication in the interpersonal setting of the group, carrying meaning for the individual, subgroup and group. Schlapobersky (1993) describes working on a dream along similar lines: [T]he dream is first a soliloquy. . . . Then it becomes the subject of a dialogue, initially between this man and his partner and then between the men and women in the group as they are all drawn into a review of their relationships. . . . [T]he group works like a chorus in an ancient drama, challenging private deceits with public recognition and confirming private recognitions with public affirmation. (p. 231) I encourage the group members to resonate to the dream 'as if it were your own'. Group members learn to emotionally resonate dreams with their personal echo and in time they are able to associate freely with the dream's narrative, which may often also represent their own emotional movements and involvements as separate individuals and as members of the group.

I propose that the first and most important 'informative' use of the dream content and its structure should be the evaluation of the dreamer's capability for exploratory or depth psychotherapy. Many participants cannot productively and progressively work (at least at the beginning) with threatening, deep interpretations or even address hidden and frightening dream aspects told in the here-and-now of the interaction following dreamtelling. Similarly, the group as a whole needs to be assessed for its readiness for this kind of work with dreams; the group needs first to go through a process of maturation and preparation for containment, during which both the dreamteller as well as the other group members need protection (Friedman, 2002b; Ullman, 1996).

Formative use of dreams

If the evaluation of the dream suggests a lack of a mature structure in its narrative, a 'formative' approach to working with the material may be needed to promote higher levels of organization in the mind of the dreamer as well as other members of the group. Rather than deep interpretation that might threaten the patient and the group, the therapist and the members may help to mould, shape, and build the shaken or fragmented self that dreamed the dream (Fosshage, 2000). Therapists too often seem indiscriminately prone to prematurely unveiling very threatening and over-exciting aspects of the dream.[3] I suggest that if the 'dream skin' is deficient, it is best developed by a non-interpretative, reinforcing dialogue that is conducive to the building of the self, as represented in the dream's structure (Anzieu, 1993). Usually, a securing interpersonal encounter is needed in which the dream's audience accompanies the dreamer and promotes the containment for the dream's anxious or exciting content. The containment of structures 'in need of mending' (Winnicott, 1969) may be done in many ways. A dream, having been told 'in the presence' of the group and just recognized without having been rejected, may already be a contribution toward the formation of a more secure transitional growing space. Also, an empathic interpersonal engagement with a dream seems to be a first containing step in the formation of a more cohesive self. Bion describes a patient so disturbed that he could only 'dream with precautions' in the presence of his psychoanalyst (1992). Retelling the dream (Friedman, 2002b) may be auxiliary in receiving external containment for unbearable and dreadful emotions. This process may be achieved by an amplification of the dream's manifest narrative, portraying details along with its accompanying feelings. A phenomenological approach to the dream can help bear the dream's experience and escort the dreamer through it. Loden (2003) describes a step-by-step formative use of the dreams of a very disturbed patient in a classical psychoanalytical setting. The self-psychology model also seems especially helpful in the formative use of dreams, by approaching dream images as expressions of affective reactions or thematic experiences rather than as the products of disguise (Stolorow et al., 2002). This non-interpretative approach may often uniquely sustain a position of empathic immersion in the patient's experience of the dream, genuinely meeting the dreamer's sense of Self and keeping in touch with threatened self-states. According to Fonagy et al. (Fonagy et al., 2002) sticking to the manifest dream without devaluation or falsification strengthens the self and promotes coherence and 'mentalization' instead of causing excessive mental pain or fears of disintegration.

Dreams told in a group which bear a fragmented character are thought to signify a warning about the dreamer's fragile state of mind or the group's current difficulties of containment. It may be advisable to just acknowledge the dream's difficult manifest content, reinforce the group's ability to tolerate difficulties, and acknowledge the courage of the group and the dreamer in order to build an elaborating partnership around the dream.

Many group therapists feel that the dream itself may be a builder of the group's mentality (Stone and Karterud, 2006; Puget, 2002). The group therapy's texture and depth may change if dreams are told, contributing to the unique way in which a group develops. Building a working culture is a core chapter in the group's growth. It seems that the self-psychology approach to dreams is particularly helpful for formative contributions, because of its sensitivity to the participants' affective shifts and vulnerability, and the protection that it offers them in their healing and developmental processes. Stone and Karterud (2006) advise us to 'look for the group's emotional responses and reactions rather than for hidden contents and interpretations' (p. 73). This approach supports a troubled dreamer in his/her containing efforts rather than pushing him/her to invest his/her energies in an exploration of his threatening and fragmenting unconscious.

In our dream vignette, it seems clear that little formative work was needed. The dream was the opposite of a fragmented dream: it was well organized and interesting, reflecting interpersonal relationships, and no depiction of catastrophic or dreadful events. However, in the interpersonal process of the dreamtelling, this dream was certainly felt as formative of the group's deeper working culture. It promoted even more security and openness about shared difficult emotions like envy, competition and dependency.

The transformative potential of dreamtelling

As posited above, telling dreams may entail both an unconscious request for containment from the other and be an effort to emotionally influence the audience (Friedman, 2002b, 2004). Dreamtelling, as the continuation of a partially unsuccessful 'mental digestion' (Bion, 1992, p. 50) started during dreaming, can be regarded as a second effort at containing. We proffer the idea that the dreamer in our vignette shares the dream with the group to further the containment of the anxieties and ambitions reflected in the dream content, primarily his enduring conflict between dependency wishes and narcissistic strivings. The dreamer's intuition resulted in his sharing the dream with the group as an (unconscious) effort to continue to 'work through the others' (Friedman, 2002b). His relationship with the group developed to a point where he started to entertain hopes that such conflicts could both be tolerated and further processed with more efficiency.

The second interpersonal, intersubjective function can be characterized by the exertion of the dreamteller's influence on the audience and their relationship. The highly cathected dream contents are not just reported but, through intersubjective processes like hidden projective and identificatory communication, effect changes in the relationship with the listeners. This dream had a strong impact on all group members: some identified strongly with certain contents. Sharing these contents led them later to openly admit to a greater closeness to the dreamer, mainly expressed by an acceptance of his needs – and more benignly reacting to his characterological flaws, especially his salient competitive urges and his narcissistic needs. This combination of emotional resonance and a developing sense of 'being part of' or 'being with' is one of the powerful and unique characteristics of group therapy.

The second interpersonal function is exemplified by achieving some progress in the dreamer's ability to be part of a relationship with the group. Telling this dream can be considered evidence of the dreamer's new openness, as well as a test of the group's acceptance of his otherness. The group participants became closer to him through their acknowledgement of his loneliness and narcissistically driven competition. While the dreamer's ambivalent relationship with me as leader angered some participants, the group ultimately developed an understanding that the dreamer was very needy of a special relationship with me, and many felt that this was the only way he knew of getting into the group: through me and by trying to give the best performance. Thus, in addition to everything that he and the group learned about interpersonal and intrapsychic processes from his dream, telling it succeeded in changing his position in the group.

Beyond the informative value of the dream, then, clinical work uses the dream material for formative and transformative ends. Therapists need to ask, What is the dreamer or the group not able to process by themselves? What is the request for containment? What is the dream's and the dreamer's impact on the relationship with the listeners? What will be the future influence of this dream? Where will the emotional movement started by the event of dreamtelling lead us?

Our dreamer's request for legitimization of his narcissistic and ambivalent place in the group is increasingly met with a degree of acceptance. The group's reactions to his dream reflect their understanding that he is unable, on his own, to elaborate his relationship with authority, and with me in particular. Listening to the dream, I feel warned about his need for 'goodness' (scouting for us), but also about his 'badness' in placing himself close to me. I recognize my own discomfort when he shows himself so open about his wish for an exclusive relationship with me, and not sensitive enough to the other members' similar wish for equal proximity to me. Initially, the group actually left him to struggle alone with his behaviour and its results, thus showing another acted-out aspect of the dream: it re-enacts loneliness, as if there is no possibility for change without involving everyone in a repetition of the patterns and emotions depicted in the dream. This may well be the essence of 'dreaming the dream' together: a dream told in the group immediately evokes a drama staged by echoes, thoughts, interpretations and resonance – in short, a discourse in which relation patterns and fantasies are not only represented but discussed and further elaborated.

The biking dream moved everyone from anger ('you are arrogant', 'you are detached' and 'you are pushy, like you push yourself') and envy ('you are manipulative of the group conductor') to compassion. The dreamer eventually achieved a better understanding of the aspects of his 'being together' with others. Different members in the group reported having had insights and better communication promoted by this dreamtelling. The associations to the story of Joseph enabled many participants to talk about their angry, rivalrous relations with siblings for parental favour. I thought that the group profited from this dream because they could let themselves be influenced by it, transitionally accepting it as if 'it were their own dream'. It was a significant step towards building a relationship in which the group and the dreamer could reciprocally trust each other's authentic emotional movement. The participant's motivations about his placement and inclusion problems were gradually contained, and the relationship changed into a competing, albeit nondestructive, linking pattern.

Summary

Dreams can profitably be conceptualized and worked with in the group as an intersubjective space in the group in which both the dreamer and the whole group (including the conductor) help to work through emotions relevant to all

(Ogden, 1996). Dreamtelling introduces a unique potential by fertilizing the associative matrix of the group and by bridging between the individual and group relations. A dream is told in a group with various parallel unconscious motivations. The group should 'dream the dream' through its collective resonance and use the new space created by the dream told to elaborate its content. The 'informative' work is usually relevant to the individual as well as to many other participants in the group, who grow through the assimilation of unique information retrieved from dreams, and to the group as a whole. Dreamtelling may be also used to 'form' and strengthen the individual's mental space and to build the group's structure. Finally, dreamtelling fulfils both the need and request for further containment from the audience as well as the desire to promote a change in the relationship between the dreamteller and his/her audience. Group members, including the conductor, should be open to the dream's elaborative aspects as well as to complementary influences on future relationships.

Notes

1 This chapter appeared previously as Friedman, R (2008) Dreamtelling as a Request for Containment – Three Uses of Dreams in Group Therapy. *International Journal of Group Psychotherapy*, Vol. 58(3): 327–344.

2 This understanding makes a further differentiation between Winnicott's two terms, 'object relating' and 'object use' (1969). For him, dreaming about someone would be 'object relating' because it is not the relation with the 'thing itself' (p. 711).

3 The reasons for this course of action are multifold: besides ignorance about the harm resulting from a premature 'plunging' interpretation (Foulkes, 1962), therapists' interventions often seem to be a countertransferential response to a challenge subliminally conveyed by the dream's content or structure.

References

Anzieu, D. (1993) The Film of the Dream. In S. Flanders (Ed.), *The Dream Discourse Today* (pp. 137–150). London and New York, NY: Routledge.

Agazarian, Y.M. (1994) The Phases of Group Development and the Systems-entered Group. In V.L. Shermer and M. Pines (Eds.), *Ring of Fire* (pp. 36–86). London: Routledge.

Bion, W.R. (1962) *Learning From Experience*. London: Heinemann.

Bion, W.R. (1992) *Cogitations*. London: Karnac.

Fonagy, P., Gergely, G., Jurist, E.L. and Target, M. (2002) *Affect Regulation, Mentalization, and the Development of the Self*. New York, NY: Other Press.

Fosshage, J.L. (2000) The Organizing Functions of Dreaming: A Contemporary Psychoanalytic Model. Commentary on paper by Hazel Ipp. *Psychoanalytic Dialogues*, 10: 103–117.

Freud, S. (1900) *The Interpretation of Dreams* (Standard Edition 4–5). London: Hogarth Press.

Friedman, R. (2000) The Interpersonal Containment of Dreams in Group Psychotherapy: A Contribution to the Work With Dreams in a Group. *Group Analysis*, 33(2): 221–234.

Friedman, R. (2002a) Developing Partnership Promotes Peace: Group Psychotherapy Experiences. *Croatian Medical Journal*, 43: 141–147.

Friedman, R. (2002b) Dream-telling as a Request for Containment in Group Therapy: The Royal Road Through the Other. In C. Neri, M. Pines and R. Friedman (Eds.), *Dreams in Group Psychotherapy* (pp. 46–67). London: Jessica Kingsley.

Friedman, R. (2004) Dreamtelling as a Request for Containment: Reconsidering the Group-analytic Approach to the Work With Dreams. *Group Analysis*, 37: 508–524.

Grotstein, J.S. (1979) Who Is the Dreamer Who Dreams the Dream and Who Is the Dreamer Who Understands It? *Contemporary Psychoanalysis*, 15: 110–169.

Grotstein, J.S. (2002) 'We Are Such Stuff as Dreams Are Made on': Annotations on Dreams and Dreaming in Bion's Works. In C. Neri, M. Pines and R. Friedman (Eds.), *Dreams in Group Psychotherapy* (pp. 110–146). London: Jessica Kingsley.

Jung, C.G. (1974) *Dreams*. Translated by R.F.C. Hull. Princeton, NJ: Princeton University Press.

Kohut, H. (1984) *How Does Analysis Cure?* Chicago, IL: University of Chicago Press.

Loden, S. (2003) The Fate of the Dream in Contemporary Psychoanalysis. *Journal of the American Psychoanalytic Association*, 51: 43–70.

Meltzer, D. (1983) *Dream–Life*. Worcester: Clunie Press.

Ogden, T.H. (1979) On Projective Identification. *International Journal of Psychoanalysis*, 60: 357–373.

Ogden, T.H. (1996) Reconsidering Three Aspects of Psychoanalytic Technique. *International Journal of Psychoanalysis*, 77: 883–900.

Puget, J. (2002) Singular Dreams: *Dreams of Link Scene and Discourse*. In C. Neri, M. Pines and R. Friedman (Eds.), Dreams in Group Psychotherapy (pp. 98–109). London: Jessica Kingsley.

Rafaelsen, L. (1996) Projections: Where Do They Go? *Group Analysis*, 29: 143–148.

Schlapobersky, J. (1993) The Language of the Group: Monologue, Dialogue and Discourse in Group Analysis. In D. Brown and L. Zinkin (Eds.), *The Psyche and the Social World: Developments in Group-analytic Theory* (pp. 211–231). London: Routledge.

Stolorow, R.D., Atwood, G.E. and Orange, D.M. (2002) *Worlds of Experience: Interweaving Philosophical and Clinical Dimensions in Psychoanalysis*. New York: Basic Books.

Stone, W. and Karterud, S. (2006) Dreams as Portraits of Self and Group Interaction. *International Journal of Group Psychotherapy*, 56: 47–61.

Ullman, M. (1996) *Appreciating Dreams: A Group Approach*. London: Sage.

Winnicott, D.W. (1969) The Use of an Object. *International Journal of Psychoanalysis*, 50: 711–716.

2

THE DREAM NARRATIVE AS AN INTERPERSONAL EVENT

Research results[1]

In psychotherapy, dreams have always been central to understanding and changing the patient. Freud (1900, 1933) stressed the intrapsychic aspects of dreaming without paying much attention to the dream narrative. But there are some important and crucial differences between dreaming and dreamtelling. This article will consider dreams from the point of view of their narrative, especially investigating the interpersonal aspects of dreamtelling in the parent-child setting. In contrast to the classical psychoanalytical intrapsychic point of view, which is interested in a dream told for the personal representation of the dreamer's unconscious, our understanding is that dreaming is an effort to (unconsciously) process overdosed threatening and exciting contents. I regard this emotional material as pertaining both to the dreamer and to significantly close Others. Thus the dreamer unconsciously takes on himself to elaborate his own as well as his environment's hardships and excitements. Moreover, I think that the dream opens the 'royal' way not only to the dreamer's inner life, in accordance with Freud's view, but also to his environment's hardships. I also propose that a dream told may represent a special opportunity to further elaborate emotions not well-enough contained. The interpersonal space created between a dreamer who tells a dream and a receptive audience that 'dreams the dream' may be an opportunity to continue an incomplete digestion process started by the dreaming event. The classic view of the dream mechanism of tension-reduction through disguise and other defences may be an explanation for the relation with the sleeping process but is not a good enough explanation for dreamtelling.

Telling dreams has an interpersonal elaborative aim: it seeks influence through potential *external* containment. This external containment is achieved through the unconscious meetings between dreamteller and dream-audience and the intersubjective process resulting from this 'encounter'. For example, a classic view of dreaming of aggressive behaviour against one's own parents may be that the dream represents the activation of destructive drives or reactions against the loved ones or a latent Oedipal conflict. But telling the dream is a (usually unconscious) communication that may potentially ignite a process of closeness and change in the character of the relationship. It may send a threatening potential as well as a request to the audience for help to contain badly controlled impulses.

A request for containment is one of the interpersonal functions of dreamtelling. It usually means that the measure of containment of the over-threatening and exciting emotions achieved by the dreaming process is not satisfactory, and an external container is sought out in order to continue the elaboration process. Telling a dream is more than the Freudian, Jungian and Kleinian contention that the dream is an event that points to potential links to unconscious and rejected parts of the Self. In addition to its contribution to the dreamer's psychic development, dreams narrated establish a link with parts of the audience Self, pushing them towards enactments and changes in their mutual future relationship. Dreamtelling has inherent Hope and even Faith (Neri, 2005), feelings which ignite internal and external processes.

Relating dreams may be considered a second step after making a first, autonomous effort to cope with overdoses of feelings. This does not mean that a dreamer's request for containment will always be an event on the edge of crisis. Often telling a dream means influencing a relationship through its contents or the quality of the dream-relation. In spite of the similarity of the contents, there is a huge difference between a patient who, close to panic, recounts that he drove his car on the road at almost breakneck speed and the adolescent who boasts that in his dream he raced his car in the city at maximum velocity. The first seeks a partner able to contain his fears regarding his impulses; the second seeks a partner who can contain his joy and pride at his (omni-)potent power. Imposing power and fears, starting a closeness process or maintaining it are but a few examples of the aims of dreamtelling.

In another example from groups, men and women may differ according to gender: women may start by telling anxious dreams in order to establish a familiar relationship through the sharing of anxieties and weakness, which results in the extension of help. Men sometimes start the dreamtelling process by sharing a dream in which the dreamer seems to be bragging, taking a (omni-)potent schizo-paranoid position and pushing to take a leading role in the group.

A person may also be a 'non-dreamer', with a Self that may not be capable of transforming beta elements into alpha thinking. The alpha function is not developed enough to 'dream' a difficulty, signifying that the individual may not be able to digest well hardships. In this case, the dream-relation may be a narrative whose main aim is to request containment. This person desperately needs another to dream his or her dream – s/he may not know how to be helped otherwise and narrates the dream with the hidden purpose of requesting containment.

Helping to narrate dreams

It follows that dreamtelling sets up developmental processes through the growth of the alpha function. The second step, containment through the Other, will of course also have its own influence on the first step: self-containment. It may be appropriate to define this kind of approach to the dream as *formative* in contrast to the more *diagnostic* approach of the classic dream theory and the subsequent *transformative* approach (Friedman, 2004). Children and patients may be forming the structure of their psyche through working on the complex unconscious sides of dreams. Considering all these different intra- and interpersonal aspects involved, it seems important to promote the dream narrative – the second, interpersonal step in the development of thinking. In order to dream, there already has to be some psychic growth, which may consist of an internalization of the parental containing (alpha) function as a prerequisite to the ability to think and cope with troublesome emotional material (Bion, 1963; Ogden, 1979). In the next stage, in order to tell dreams, there has to be the feeling that a relationship can contain the dreams told. While dreaming as a mental activity seems to be quite independent of remembering dreams, 'dreaming' as a digestive coping activity is not an automatic quality that everyone has (Ogden, 1996; Grotstein, 1979; Bion, 1992). If it does not develop naturally, external help is needed. Bion made the remark about a psychotic patient, that he 'could only dream in the presence of his analyst' (ibid, p. 40).

There seems to be a strong interconnection between dreamtelling and dream-listening. This link is evident to therapists who discover, along with their patients, that a therapeutic relationship that is open to the unconscious promotes both dream-remembering and the narrative of dreams. Even patients who report 'not to dream' are surprised when they start therapy by a spontaneous 'new' ability to connect through dreams to their inner world. I believe such a development cannot be the result of suggestion alone. Elsewhere (Friedman, 2002a) I speculated about the nature of remembering dreams: it is connected with the presence of a container for dreams. This container may be a significant relationship that is able to tolerate and even be interested in the world represented in the dream. For many this is the precursor of relationships that help bear and elaborate the hardship of 'dream life' (Meltzer, 1983). Moreover, I think (Friedman, 2003b) that before there is a chance to introject this external container, a 'moment of meeting' between a panic-stricken child who has an overwhelming nightmare and his receptive parents establishes a special kind of relationship. The child cries out, requesting containment from his genitors, the 'container-on-call', who join in an elaborating partnership in order to bear the emotional difficulties of the dream. In spite of the fact that such a relationship begins through a mostly non-verbal interaction, this first imprintive episode contributes to an ability to use dreams personally and interpersonally. It may promote both the 'dreaming' of the first stage as an effort for autonomous containment and the following second stage of dreamtelling. This sequela makes it possible to complete a not-good-enough oneiric elaboration through external containment. Thus dreamtelling may have learned components initially acquired in a nightly environment.

Furthermore, I draw several conclusions from clinical observations: one is that men are not at all good containers for dreams and that women have difficulties containing male dreams. This observation points to difficulties in parental containment, which makes it difficult for the development of elaborating partnerships for dreams. Fathers seem to be not-good-enough containers for dreams. Mothers may have fewer difficulties containing their sons' dreams as they can be good at bearing them (for a while only), but not at elaborating them. As a result, parents generally are not able to really digest and return the better digested material to their children. Containing reinforces and supports dreamtelling; non-containment extinguishes it. Men do not like to cope with or share threatening contents of dreams, especially if they are opposed to the normative male roles of power and strength. Dreams that expose the dreamer as being panic-stricken, victimized, or avoiding male tasks and assuming female tasks are very difficult to bear, but are dreamt by everyone. Mothers, basically more apt and able to contain many dreams, are much better equipped to bear and elaborate their daughter's dreams than their son's nightmares. This lack of containment of the boy's dreams is learned from both parents and usually starts a reenactment of men's inability to work through many emotional difficulties. This line of thought has led me to investigate dreamtelling patterns in the family, an endeavour still in process.

Investigating dream contents in children

For this purpose, we formulated a questionnaire at Haifa University comprising 21 questions. Investigations of the *dream contents* of children found that there are significant developments in children's dreams (Ram, 1997) Five-year-old children dream longer than younger children and have a greater ability to describe the background of their dreams. This is in line with the development of the ego's abilities to 'think', e.g. work through difficulties. There are also significant gender differences reflected by the dream contents. Both genders 'dream' about the emotions and the preoccupations of daily interpersonal situations, even more than adults do. But boys and girls differ significantly in the level and quality of aggressive contents dreamt. Boys dream of more powerful activity and significantly more physical violence than girls do, equivalent to the quotidian games they play. In contrast to girls, who more often dream themselves as victims, boys also tend to distance themselves from victimized representation, preferring to dream of hurt animals rather than humans, especially close ones.

Investigating dreamtelling

Continuing this line of investigation, I found, like many of my colleagues in clinical practice, that there are significant gender differences in dreamtelling. The difference in contents may be one element responsible for the fact that men tell fewer dreams than females do. We tried to investigate the relationship between container (the parental audience) and contained (the child dreamer) that is hypothetically responsible for the extinction or evocation of dream narrative. This investigation focused on the establishment of an elaborative dialogue, the 'working-through' partnership (Friedman, 2002a). It seems possible to apply the narrative abilities of dreams together with their elaboration to specific areas, like coping with male domestic violence and the relationship abilities of females. Apparently, females' abilities to narrate their emotional difficulties via saturated communicative channels, like dreams, promote the growth of their social skills. On the other hand, we might say that the lack of elaborative spaces like dreamtelling preserves the potential for violence in men. Perhaps such deficient development is unconsciously promoted by the society that profits from primitive aggression, using non-elaborate belligerence for the community's own protection.

In previous investigations we found that children's dreamtelling is not different for boys and girls until about the fifth year. Men's dreamtelling makes a relative comeback when men court or are in love. We searched for evidence that boys' dreamtelling is extinguished or at least negatively reinforced somewhere in early childhood. We also looked for evidence that women get support for their dreamtelling by a positive environmental (especially parental) response. In individual and group therapy we can easily observe an influence of the therapeutic space generating a diminishment or augmentation of dreamtelling in both men and women

Research on dreamtelling in the family

Ninety-five questionnaires were validated in which parents were asked about gender differences in dreams related by their children. They were also asked about differences in their responses to the boys' and girls' dreams and about similarities between the child's tendency to tell a dream and the parent's own history of dreamtelling.

Only 10 men answered in contrast to 85 women. The parents' mean age was 43. They averaged 15 years of education and came mostly from the north of Israel.

Results

In this investigation there was no evidence that boys told fewer dreams to their mothers than girls did. Interestingly, there was significant evidence that girls told more dreams to their fathers than boys did.

There were differences concerning the content of dreams: boys told significantly more nightmares, while girls told more 'pleasant' dreams. However, there seemed to be more interpretative responses to boys' than to the girls' dreams. This investigation corroborates the accepted finding that men remember and report significantly fewer dreams than women do.

Conclusion

Most of the findings provide evidence for the basic assumption that dreamtelling is an acquired interpersonal event. The difference in the dreamtelling of nightmares may be connected to the different interpersonal socialization of boys and girls. Boys' dreams reveal that they have to cope with more overt, and overtly physical, aggression and seem to work hard at night to try and work these excitements through.

The inherent difficulties in succeeding to do so may be one of the factors that inhibit the memory of dreams. This investigation produced no clear results about why there is a significant difference in dreamtelling.

We can assume that the difference in the dream contents will have a differential impact on the audience. Findings about men remembering and telling significantly fewer dreams than women may lead to the assumption that the availability of a container influenced the memory of dreams and thus the use of dream narratives as a further instrument of elaboration. Something in the boys' past seems to have extinguished dream-remembering and dreamtelling.

We have the feeling that the questionnaires were not accurate enough to establish and understand gender differences. For example, although we know that boys' dreamtelling diminishes after the age of five to seven (for whatever reasons), there was no significant trace of such a development in the results. The finding that girls tell more dreams to their fathers than boys do is to be taken with a grain of salt (because of the low number of fathers asked) but leads to interesting speculations. Essentially, the difference strengthens the assumptions that dreamtelling is an interpersonal event. Boys, regardless of the reason, have more difficulties telling their dreams to their parents, and their role as 'male' overtakes every other aspect. This result is in line with the hypothesis that men do not like to cope with 'male' dreams – and as fathers, they certainly prefer their daughters' dreams. Maybe this preference is more for the attachment to their daughters than for the dream contents. The daughter-father bond may be strengthened by being able to contain dreams, while the fathers' containment of their sons seems to be lacking. This finding should be further investigated with a greater number of fathers and deeper quality research of their containment.

Applications for everyday life

These results may contribute to the awareness that many men with a very rich internal life do not tell their dreams because of a faulty interpersonal experience. If we wish to restore the ability to communicate the internal life and re-establish contact with men's unconscious in order to further promote development, we have to build a container that facilitates access to the dreamer's ability to share and work through difficult contents. This can be done at any age, but it seems to be easiest if parents are helped by teaching them to provide a container for the dream narration. Men in particular do not have the necessary skills to promote containment in their children. Perhaps specifically it is the boys' dreams that are especially difficult to contain. Recently, we have had mothers in groups that have learned to cope with their boys' violence in dreams. This is done through understanding the dynamics of dreaming and dreamtelling through reciprocal reflection on dreams narrated. In addition, exposure to films with violent contents (like Dogville, 2003) are instrumental in exploring and facilitating the communication of inner violence, which allows the link and containment between mothers and their children's aggression.

Note

1 This chapter appeared previously as Friedman, R (2006a) The dream narrative as an interpersonal event – research results. *funzionegamma*. La Sapienza, University of Rome.

References

Bion, W. (1963) *Elements of Psycho-Analysis*. London: Jason Aronson.

Bion, W. (1992) *Cogitations*. London: Karnac.

Freud, S. (1900) *The Interpretation of Dreams* (Standard Edition 4–5). London: Hogarth Press.

Freud, S. (1933) *New Introductory Lectures on Psycho-Analysis* (Standard Edition 22). London: Hogarth Press

Friedman, R. (2002a) Developing Partnership Promotes Peace: Group Psychotherapy Experiences. *Croatian Medical Journal*, 43(2): 141–147.

Friedman, R. (2002b) Dream-Telling as a Request for Containment in Group Therapy: The Royal Road Through the Other. In M. Pines, C. Neri and R. Friedman (Eds.), *Dreams in Group Psychotherapy*. London: Jessica Kingsley Publishers.

Friedman, R. (2004) Dreamtelling as a Request for Containment – Reconsidering the Group-Analytic Approach to the Work With Dreams. *Group Analysis*, 37(4): 508–524.

Grotstein, J.S. (1979) Who Is the Dreamer Who Dreams the Dream and Who Is the Dreamer Who Understands It? *Contemporary Psychoanalysis*, 15(1).

Meltzer, D. (1983) *Dream-Life*. Worcester: Clunie Press.

Neri, C. (2005) What Is the Function of Faith and Trust in Psychoanalysis. *International Journal of Psychoanalysis*, 86: 79–97.

Ogden, T.H. (1979) On Projective Identification. *International Journal of Psychoanalysis*, 60: 357–373.

Ogden, T.H. (1996) Reconsidering Three Aspects of Psychoanalytic Technique. *International Journal of Psychoanalysis*, 77(5): 883–900.

Ram, O. (1997) *The Comparison of Different Themes and Aggressive Patterns as Appearing in Dreams and Free Play of Four-to-Six Year Old Children*. Unpublished Paper, Thesis submitted at the University of Haifa.

von Trier, L. (2003) *Dogville*. Lions Gate Films.

3

USING THE TRANSPERSONAL IN DREAMTELLING AND CONFLICT[1,2]

Introduction

Group analysis is a uniquely helpful therapeutic modality, sometimes complementing other therapies. What makes it an optimal approach for promoting the health and development of individuals and communities? It provides a space where individuals and subgroups may achieve what cannot be done alone or in dyads, and allows for special contents to emerge. It arouses unique emotional states and it is a field that enables unique emotional movements. The group's emotional 'traffic' between participants depends on their courage and openness and the conductor's skill.

Group-analytic groups provide optimal opportunity for such interpersonal 'traffic' (Foulkes, 1975: 253) by the transpersonal, a special quality of communication enabled by a heightened permeability between the participants' Selves. It makes it possible to work with others and through others. Through becoming aware of the communication flow in the group, members develop higher abilities to participate in the interpersonal space. They learn to see and use the transpersonal, enhancing the quality of their interactions. It can be exemplified by a person who stands in the dark, but is given a NVD[3] that suddenly enables him to 'see' both others and themselves. This heightened vision provides understanding of the social space and a greater ability to navigate relationships in a more positive way, together with a greater awareness of his or her life.

Group analysis makes a differentiation between the transpersonal and the interpersonal. Foulkes and Anthony say that 'In further formulation of our observation we have come to conceive these processes *not merely as interpersonal* but as *transpersonal*' (1957: 26). It means that the transpersonal is different from an interpersonal communication by being both a communication between people but mainly 'through' them, using their psyche. Using the transpersonal provides individuals the tools to investigate and change the ways in which they belong to groups. It also allows them to cope with rejection and exclusion anxiety, which are fundamental human relational emotions and pervade, with different degrees of awareness, all social situations. Learning to use the transpersonal enables group-analytic group participants to investigate interpersonal emotional movement, like seeking recognition and influence. The interpersonal sphere is the space in which human interactions happen – the transpersonal aspect is the mode in which to understand interactions. '[T]ranspersonal phenomena goes to the very roots of any approach to group psychology and requires a *fundamental turn of mind*' (Foulkes, 1964: 18).

Nitzgen (2010) thinks the transpersonal connects us to the symbolic register (personal communication); it is an abstraction, which goes beyond the manifest communication. In a day-to-day reality, it also enables many ways of individual participants using one another, for example, by telling each other their dreams. The group-analytic group is the dancing floor on which this unique transpersonal movement takes place – it is an invitation for deep richness to create together and to dream together. (And people have to be invited to dance.)

The late Yehuda Amihai, an Israeli poet, captured the essence of group analysis, when he wrote:

> People use each other
> As a healing for the pain. They put each other
> on their existential wounds,
> on eye, on mouth and open hand.
> They hold each other hard and won't let go
> *(Amihai, 1986: 77)*

In group analysis we are aware that while the notion *transpersonal* is quite similar, if not identical, to the 'relational' intersubjective, it nonetheless precedes it by a generation (Friedman, 2014). In 1954, Foulkes described interpersonal psychodynamics as 'transpersonal manifestations' that do not 'confine (themselves) within the boundaries of the individual but regularly include a number of interconnected persons' (1954: 26). This approach was taken up more than 30 years later when Mitchell described the relational matrix as 'the most useful way to view psychological reality . . . as encompassing both intrapsychic and interpersonal realms' (1988: 9). The concepts of the transpersonal and the matrix may also facilitate a closer dialogue with the relational approach in psychoanalysis.

I understand the term *transpersonal* to refer to the unique permeable way in which participants of a group-analytic group relate among themselves, 'an endopsychic common union between . . . people' (Foulkes, 1966: 154). In a matrix, transpersonal connections are processes which 'go through the individuals – similar to X-rays in the physical sphere' (Foulkes, 1973: 229).

The permeable boundaries of the mind enable 'concerts of interactions' and make for the 'transpersonal character' of relations. Transpersonal processes are contagious, influential and include introjections, projections and 'projective identifications' (Redl, 1942; Rafaelsen, 1996).[4]

Applying the concept of 'transpersonality' to our practice, I will expand the transpersonal approach to the unconscious communicative dream-life in the matrix. The group-analytic approach also suggests a shift in our understanding of pathological relationships (Friedman, 2007, 2013), which will not be discussed in this chapter. Finally, I shall refer to applications of group-analytic thinking in the field of conflict resolution.

The uses of dreams in group analysis: dreaming and dreamtelling as a request for containment

The same transpersonal principles which are used to define healthy and pathologic relations, which include psychic permeability, reciprocal influence in the social unconscious matrix, and strong intersubjective valency, are applied once again to the realm of dreaming and dreamtelling.

Since Artemidorus from Daldia, who was the first to write 'The Interpretation of Dreams' (third century BCE, cited in White, 1990), and certainly since Freud (1900), many accept that the contents of our dreams, as well as the processes of dreaming, reveal the essence and secrets of our minds. Why are there so many apparent difficulties to make good use of our dreams, while acknowledging that dreams represent our vast inner wealth? Why does Shakespeare wish dreams would fade away, 'leave not a rack (a wisp of cloud) behind? (*The Tempest*)'. It seems that our 'True Self' (Winnicott, 1965) and its unique and creative reflection in dreams and nightmares is paradoxically too overwhelming and too frightening to bear. Hanna Segal states ambivalently: 'the structure of the dream reflects the structure of personality' (1993: 100). It may be often shameful and painful to acknowledge 'the stuff we are made on' (Shakespeare). Dreaming and dreamtelling, embedded in the transpersonal approach of group analysis, may stimulate new ways to understand and elaborate both contents and messages of dreams. This approach is not exclusive, but it goes beyond the intrapersonal or individual contents of dreams shifting to the understanding that interpersonal aspects are part and parcel of the work of dreams and every dream told. The transpersonal enriches the elaboration of dreams by the differentiation of three uses of dreamtelling: an informative, a formative and an approach (or use) which changes relations, the transformative use of dreams.

Informative approach

Example

Here is an example of a fragment of a dream, which I will refer to again later:

> I walk to my mother with a tray of marbles. I want her to see them.

There is already quite a lot of *information* in the dream. Freud and many of his followers, such as Klein, Bion and others would have looked for hidden meanings to the manifest contents like 'approaching mother', 'marbles' and 'the wish to be seen'. This effort I have called the *informative approach* (Friedman, 2006, 2012). Interpreting dreams' contents is still considered the 'royal way' to retrieve information of the dreamer's psychodynamics, his relation to the group and to the therapist. The task of understanding dreams has become one of the most fascinating elements of our trade. Every generation and group of psychoanalysts have developed aspects of the work with dreams: discerning hidden feelings in dream contents, diagnosing the dreamer, the group, and gaining a deeper understanding about the dreamer's splits into the 'me' parts of the dream and 'not-me' parts, etc. The understanding that those we are connected with are part of the dreams, their meaning and their purpose, has made many other perspectives on dreams possible.

Do we only dream for ourselves?

Dreaming may be less of an exclusive personal function than we believe. The *transpersonal* perspective suggests that an individual's dreaming function may be 'used' (Winnicott, 1971) by partners, children, spouses, patients and groups to process their emotional difficulties. Dreaming is an elaborating and containing process (Bion, 1992; Ogden, 1996; Friedman, 2002, 2012) function, which digests excessive threats and excitements. The dreaming abilities of one person may also be unconsciously used by those close to him to contain transpersonal conflicts and transgenerational traumas and other difficulties – in the same way as Bion (1962) shows how mothers process, through their alpha function, their children's overwhelming emotions, the unthinkable beta elements. Therapists and patients may use their processing function, their dreaming, reciprocally. Accordingly, we may immediately have an additional perspective to our understanding of the dream in our example: does 'showing the marbles' represent the dreamer's infantile need (a classic approach to dreams) or does it also represent the dreamer's effort to satisfy his mother's constant need for narcissistic supplies? The dream may be dreamt to calm the mother.

To further deepen our understanding of dreaming and dreamtelling: they may be considered as two consecutive and complementary steps in the process of emotional elaboration. Dreaming seems to be a first effort to process individually an excessive emotion, potentially followed by a second processing effort through dreamtelling. Remembering a dream and then sharing it in a transpersonal matrix in order to elaborate it can usually be done on the condition that the dreamer has or had a suitable partner.[5] Then dreamtelling may bring us a step further in the elaboration of difficult feelings by re-dreaming the dream 'through the Other'. In our short example, the dreamer alone may not be able to reach further elaboration of his and his mother's needs without dreamtelling, sharing his dream with a partner who is willing to even unconsciously participate in the containment of the dream's contents and messages.

Dreamtelling starts non-verbally when an infant cries out in his dream, requesting containment. If he meets a 'container-on-call' (that is, a parent who keeps him in his mind and rushes to his/her bed) a potential partnership may be facilitated for life. Investigating 90 women and 90 men for their family history of dream-sharing, at Haifa University we found support for the notion that 'where there is a container there is dreamtelling' and vice versa (Dayan, 2010). It means first that containing relationships influence both our memory and the will to share. This research also validates the importance of parental ability to address dreamtelling in families and groups as a valuable element of communication.

Transformation of relations through dreamtelling

A further use of dreamtelling's transpersonal social potential is to consider dreams as a communication that 'transforms relationships'. The dreamer in our example influences us, the listeners, to touch similar conscious and unconscious emotional positions he felt and shared in his dream: we almost immediately share his feeling of wanting to show mother the marbles – it spills into showing us, the audience, his dream and changes the atmosphere of the relation by this same emotional movement represented in the dream: trying to establish a relationship by presenting something.

Dreamtelling is actualized and amplified in group-analytic groups, which together with the conductor create a space in which dreams can resonate through other members rather than through interpretation. Personal and group insights and the *informative* function are deepened by sharing the group's spontaneous individual affective responses – the personal resonance reflecting (unconscious) identifications with latent contents. This resonance travels like transpersonal 'X-rays' between dreamers and listeners to dreams. This approach to dreams enables *transformative* processes because it creates 'moments of meetings' (Stern et al., 1998) that change the relations between dreamtellers and the dreamlisteners who engage in 'dreaming the dreams'. Thus resonance to dreamtelling is not a simple emotional echo, but furthers elucidation and elaboration of the dream told through transpersonal re-dreaming. Interpreting too fast may rather dissociate the interpreters from the dreamer, the dream and its multilevel influences on the relation between all involved, and should be allowed to happen later in the process. In an effort to facilitate the emotional conscious and unconscious echo to the dreamtelling event, when a dream is told in a group for the first time, I usually ask members to 'try and listen to the dream as though it was your own. Try to relate to it through your own life-experience and let us hold off interpretations for later'. Groups more often than not learn this 'language' and allow a less defensive communication with a dreamer and his dream.

Example continued

To return to the dream in my example:

In a group-analytic group Marco, a male participant (39) who joined some months before, told his first dream:

I want to tell a dream I already told in individual therapy about a year ago. I walk to my mother with a tray of marbles. I want her to see them. She is dressed in a blue, elegant outfit surrounded by friends, men and women. She whispers something to a man. Then she turns around and walks away. I try to follow her but trip over the foot of the man, and the marbles scatter all over the floor. The man steps on them and says to me: 'Let's go to the toilet'.

Anna (57): It hurt me in my belly. It reminds me of my father's cold and denigrating reactions to me.

Belinda (30): I think your mother was very intimate with this man. . . . [S]he double-crossed you!

Therapist: Belinda: Do you say this because of your own life-experience? Where did it touch you?

Belinda: My mother always considered men and work to be more important than us.

Carl (45): For me, there was something sexually exciting. I'm a bit ashamed to say this, but there is dirty sex in the air. It's even frightening; yesterday in a bar with my wife and some friends I couldn't stop watching a young girl, who could be my child, who I wanted to go to the toilet with.

David (62): I'm amazed of what I remembered when I heard the dream: I would come home from school and have a nap with my mother until I was 10 or more. I was sure that my mother would always want to nap with me, for as long as I wanted it.

Elaine (42): I feel terrible . . . (long pause). Everything I didn't want to think about came back to me: my uncle inviting me to have a nap with him, my grandfather forcing me to sit on his lap, my former friend forcing himself on me. . . . I cannot avoid talking about it anymore.

As usual, after a while I came back to the dreamer to ask if the group members' responses rang any bells. He was extremely moved by emotions he had not felt, and insights that he had not understood before. His individual therapist tried to give meaning to the marbles and 'going together to the toilet'. But the sexuality, his desire to conquer his mother, her rejection and his seductiveness had not been touched upon. His mother had felt very close to him, and he now wondered about the boundaries between them.

Elaine: Maybe she did this to protect you? In my own family there was no such protection. Older relatives could abuse a girl and everyone would turn a blind eye.

Belinda shares with the group her willingness to do everything for a man who is good to her. It is so important to feel wanted.

I ask the group if our intimacy has become so strong that hidden wishes and worries threaten the boundaries. Do we need more security and protection? The question seems to help the group to re-join the work, communicating formerly unspoken thoughts and feelings, which echo the dream, unconsciously informing this dreamer and his past, present and future relations. Through this I propose a connection between the dreamer, his dream and the wish to change the relation to our group.

The dreamer's request for containment and demand for influence

Introducing this dream into the permeable mind of the transpersonal matrix, can help to unravel hidden emotional messages in the group while also igniting a working-through process of many of the participators who allow themselves to be touched by resonating with the dream, as if it was their own.

I used to ask myself two questions which go beyond informative work to the transformative aspects of this dreamtelling: (1) What is the dreamer's request for containment in (from?) the group? and (2) What is the influence the dreamer is seeking from (on) the audience? I think this dreamer requests containment (Friedman, 2002) (of) his fears of rejection, which he cannot contain alone. He is willing to give a lot, to show his marbles in order to avoid exclusion, often overpaying a price to become central in groups as a defence against feelings of loneliness, inferiority and fear of rejection. He cannot cope with envy and aggression and asks the group to help him out of the perpetrator/victim role connection. While it seems important to try to understand the significance of the marbles or of the toilet, it seems to me equally important to be aware of the emotional movement in the group stimulated by the dream.

So, I started to address the fears of exclusion introduced by this extremely boundary-less dreamer, who, as in his defensive patterns, had seduced the group to enormous intimacy. This kind of transpersonal emotional traffic in the matrix may both attract and frighten the group because of the unconscious pull to re-enact latent dream patterns. Dreams contain powerful feelings, which may be able to move the audience beyond awareness even to action. Here, in our example, participants felt that they would possibly want to exclude and to reject this dreamer. The request for containment in a dream is part of the *transformative* use of dreamtelling. It is transformative because the elaboration by others opens some further emotional and behavioural possibilities for the dreamer, but also because it changes the relations with the audience. Those listening to the dream will share the encounter with the excessively threatening or exciting emotions aroused by the dream.

Dreams told have a past, they voice a present and create a future. Thus in the sessions after the dream is told, therapists should be alert to changes in relationships in the group which are a development caused by the dreamtelling.

After a while the dreamer said that the group had opened a whole new world for him by reacting to his dream. In these moments, the group looks like the optimal place to explore both unconscious meanings and their transpersonal impact on relationships. Giving dreams a place in analysis enabled Belinda two sessions later to say that the dream helped her to understand how her expressed neediness while looking for a job would intensify people's feelings of rejection.

Dreamtelling facilitates work *with others and through others* using transpersonal processes that make *informational* work deeper and transformation of emotions and relations possible. Transpersonal relating is instrumental to obtaining and containing personal insights from the dream told; thus it is an important contribution to the *informative use of dreams.*

Does this approach to the group's elaboration of the unconscious, by first resonating emotionally and only later conceptualizing the process, challenge the notion of freedom of association? Group-analytic patients may feel freer when they are somewhat better contained and protected by the conductor and the setting. Participators are able then to engage in resonating the dreamtelling, thus working in the group in a more liberated form, possibly making it unnecessary for the dreamer to opt for processing his dream in an individual therapeutic setting, which often gives the illusion of being better protected. It is also possible for the conductor to feel a different personal emotional response to the dreamer's and the group's request for containment and protection (see also Ullman, 1996). In our case, the conductor felt a great need to protect the dreamer, which he shared with others in the group.

The formative approach

The third use of dreamtelling, the *formative approach*, results from the clinical experience that interpretations frighten some dreamers, or may cause them and the relations in the group more damage than good. The therapist should be able to have instruments that enable a clinical choice between an explorative and a supportive approach to dreams, which voice some of the excessively threatening and exciting emotions. When working with dreamers who are children, psychotic, etc. and sometimes immature patients, the therapist may prefer to work in a supportive, non-interpretative way. If the dreamer's Self is damaged, fragmented or just not developed enough it should be first strengthened, or 'formed' by supportive interventions. The support may include re-telling (even after months), repeating, drawing and rewriting the dream's manifest contents. Repairing his 'dream skin-ego' (Anzieu, 1993) by a *formative* approach re-structures 'the stuff we are made on'. Instead of 'exploration', the therapist and the group first connect to the dreamer, as if accompanying the dreamer through the detailed narrative of the dream (Loden, 2003). This approach slowly develops a more resilient Self. Working formatively with the dreams of the young or with borderlines or patients in danger of disintegration may often be the optimal approach. How do we evaluate dreams in order to know how to intervene? Some security can be attained by evaluating the strength of the relations with the dreamer and the dreamer's Self. It is also possible to get some measure of security by looking into the dream's contents: if the narrative is more or less coherent and includes some humans or movement, chances are that a *formative* approach is not needed and the dream may be met, encountered and then interpreted. Working *formatively* by listening, accompanying the dreamer and the group through fears threatening affective moments as if grabbing an infant's hand through a dark ally, engenders the most powerful 'moments of meetings' (Stern et al., 1998), which enhances therapy significantly. Groups must also be sometimes helped to go along with the dreamer's pace of development and rather refrain from interpretations.

Applying group analysis when meeting the enemy?

The transpersonal has affected our work with dreams as well as the conceptualization of an interpersonal pathology or relation disorders (Friedman, 2007, 2013). A third area of application of the transpersonal is group work in conflict dialogues (sometimes called 'reconciliation'). This work is done in three areas: the best known is negotiations between decision makers in small or median groups. The second area consists of conflict dialogue between groups who seem to be under similar emotional pressure but do not have the power to decide, e.g. think tanks, politicians and civil society workers who 'meet the enemy'. Encounters of this kind happen more often than we think in different settings, including conferences and working parties. There are teams of Israelis and Palestinians who negotiate the shared handling of water, or the mental health of traumatized women. All these groups usually go through extremely difficult conflicts, even the group who met to create the Oslo agreement.

Finally, a third area for conflict dialogue that has to elaborate constantly strong emotions is the meeting between groups of civilians or sides in the conflict who could be helped to 'live' better with each other if they could improve their relationship. Meeting rivals and developing a dialogue with them may often be the best and only long-term solution to decades and centuries of animosity and hate. Even in regions that have achieved legal and political agreements between leaders – e.g. Northern Ireland – there seems to be a necessity to elaborate 'unfinished business' of enmity engendered feelings in order to achieve peace.

In this third area, pre- and post-agreement efforts have to be worked through in different settings. Often large-scale settings will be possible to apply, which may include the use of a combination of small, median and large groups. In order to make significant meetings possible, parties have to go through a sometimes painful process of lowering the defences, which the societies have used in a war matrix. While being under threat, there is a natural tendency to disengage and dissociate from the hated or feared enemy in order to *reduce transpersonal* influences. Distancing, disengaging and dissociating are among the strongest defences against a relational, intersubjective or transpersonal communication. Its major outcome is a significant reduction of feelings of guilt, shame and empathy, which are aggression-inhibiting feelings. Thus the relational disengagement seems functional to make fighting easier; recruiting the population to the war effort by a counter-identification with the enemy, encourages monolithic thinking powerful identification with the (war) matrix, which I call the soldiers' matrix (Friedman, 2013). In meetings and negotiations, transpersonal engagement is initially always met with resistance. It is as if we all know unconsciously that in times of war, avoiding the enemy creates an immunization to aggression-inhibiting emotions; serious negotiations are jeopardized through hate and avoidance. Relations seem to make fighting difficult.

In all three settings the moving from a 'flight/fight' position to less defensive positions is difficult but possible. Conductors, who have themselves gone through the process from hate to dialogue, and a protecting setting can provide the support needed during such a process.

In the IDI[6] we learned some of these processes through our efforts to bridge gaps between the West and Islam. For some of us, personal experiences in confrontational talks with Palestinians (Friedman, 2010, 2014) were transformational. Changing from an active, non-reflective participant in violence to being a human being willing to bear the pain, hate, frustration (and satisfaction) of the 'dialoguing stance' needs model leaders. Prime Minister Rabin's modelling transformation from being a fighting soldier to agreeing to shake Arafat's hand on the lawn of the White House is certainly a milestone in the development of many individuals, certainly in my own. It mirrors a potential change. It also requires encounters, which mix the personal and the large group identity (Volkan, 2006) in a mixed setting of small and large groups.

Encountering Palestinians became for me, after some months, one of the most painful processes I had ever experienced. It took more months of listening to each other's suffering, which filled us with guilt, shame and frustration for a long time, until some joy and humanity also entered the relationship. Some of the professionals from Palestine whom we met refused to share any guilt with us. Even as suicide bombers were exploding in our streets, killing hundreds, our Palestinian partners continued to battle the 'war on guilt'. The Israeli subgroup had to contain and elaborate these issues, especially by differentiating between real guilt and fantasized guilt feelings. Overcoming the blame of 'betraying' family and friends was also a difficult emotional process, which was tackled in the talks with Israelis and later Palestinians.

In the IDI we struggle for awareness of social and affective positions that affect political processes; we believe it is not possible to ignore the impact of transgenerational heritage, which functions through transpersonal principles. Emotional communicative permeability between related people makes transgenerational transmission of feelings, traumas and emotional positions possible. Thus the transpersonal principle influences the work with guilt, hate, fear and pride as well as their 'sudden' disappearance in the face of perceived threats. Dialogues and negotiations should use emotions to conceptualize the enormous energies involved and also move from what 'should be' to 'how things are'.

Not only do emotions have to be taken into account, but it is often useful to understand the deeper transpersonal impact in the dialogue with the enemy. Together with the importance of understanding the dynamics inside the matrix, there is a necessity to understand how enemy-soldiers matrices unconsciously affect and influence each other, as permeable transpersonal related organisms do. In this endeavour, I am also helped by dreams, which often hold the wisdom to acknowledge personal and social realities through exposing active 'not me' aspects I wish to deny.

During the recent conflict between Israel and Hamas (August 2014) I tried very hard to keep my 'thinking' abilities alive – different to the processes many of my fellow countrymen went through, who were feeling totally identified with the government's activity. I tried to keep thinking on questions such as what does Hamas 'really' want, what might be the alternatives under the threat of more rockets, etc. I tried to distance myself from mainstream Israeli opinions. I consider distancing oneself from one's own large group identity to be an important individuation process necessary in different meetings with the enemy e.g. in order to negotiate sincerely with neighbours. Such a separation can be achieved by participation in large groups, in order to cope with annihilation anxieties and other well-established defences against individuation.

But the night before a difficult meeting with people who had conflicting positions and adverse feelings, I had the following dream: I was fighting in long trenches between young soldiers who were running in a long row, shooting and aiming quite differently to how I had once learned it. I was concerned about being out of date, and afraid of falling down and disturbing the whole attack. I woke up sweating and feeling anxious.

While there are many valid interpretations to the dream, it struck me that the dream represented a re-identification with the soldiers' matrix. The threat of war enlists everyone in society: fighting men and women alike, and the old and the young.

Notes

1 This chapter appeared previously as Friedman, R. (2015) Using the Transpersonal in Dream-telling and Conflict. *Group Analysis*, 48(1), 1–16.
2 Based on a lecture in the London Symposium 2011: 'New Developments in group analysis'.
3 Night Vision Device.
4 Raphaelson considered projective identification one of 'the most important communicative tools' in groups.
5 Research in families showed that growing up with containing partners may enable dreaming and dreamtelling potentials. Early – good and bad – experiences with partnership elaboration while dreamtelling influence the handling of dreams for life (Dayan, 2010).
6 An organization devoted to the investigation and resolution of conflicts, especially to the encounter between the West and Islam. www.internationaldialoginitiative.com

References

Amihai, Y. (1986) *Love Poems* (A Bilingual Edition, pp. 77–78). Tel Aviv: Schocken.

Anzieu, D. (1993) The Film of the Dream. In S. Flanders (Ed.), *The Dream Discourse Today* (pp. 137–150). London and New York: Routledge.

Artemidorus Daldianus (1975) *Oneirocritica: The Interpretation of Dreams*. Translated and commented by R.J. White. Park Ridge, NJ: Noyes Press. Original Books.

Bion, W.R. (1962) *Learning From Experience*. London: Heinemann.

Bion, W.R. (1992) *Cogitations*. London: Karnac.

Dayan, D. (2010) *Relationship Between Interfamily Childhood Dream Telling Patterns and of Adulthood Dream Telling Patterns*. Unpublished Master Thesis, Haifa University, Haifa.

Foulkes, S.H. (1954) Group Processes and the Individual in the Therapeutic Group. In S.H. Foulkes (Ed.), (1964) *Therapeutic Group Analysis* (p. 180). Originally in *British Journal of Medical Psychology*, 34: 23–31.

Foulkes, S.H. (1966) Some Basic Concepts in Group Psychotherapy. In E. Foulkes (Ed.), *Selected Papers* (pp. 155–158). London: Karnac.

Foulkes, S.H. (1973) The Group as Matrix of the Individual's Mental Life. In E. Foulkes (Ed.), *Selected Papers* (pp. 223–234). London: Karnac.

Foulkes, S.H. (1975) *Group Analytic Psychotherapy: Method and Principles.* London: Gordon and Breach. Reprinted London: Maresfield, Karnac, 1986.

Foulkes, S.H. and Anthony, J. (1957) *Group Psychotherapy: The Psychoanalytic Approach.* London: Penguin, Harmondsworth. Reprinted London: Maresfield, Karnac Books, 1989.

Freud, S. (1900) *The Interpretation of Dreams* (Standard Edition 4–5). London: Hogarth Press.

Friedman, R. (2002) Dream-Telling as a Request for Containment in Group Therapy – The Royal Road Through the Other. In M. Pines, C. Neri and R. Friedman (Eds.), *Dreams in Group Psychotherapy* (pp. 46–67). London: Jessica Kingsley Publishers.

Friedman, R. (2006) Who Contains the Group and Who Is the Leader? A Relational Disorders Perspective. *European Journal of Psychotherapy* (EJPCH Group Edition), 8(1): 21–32.

Friedman, R. (2007) Where to Look? Supervising Group Analysis – A Relations Disorder Perspective. *Group Analysis* 40(2): 251–268.

Friedman, R. (2010) The Group and the Individual in Conflict and War. *Group Analysis*, 43(3): 281–300.

Friedman, R. (2012) Dreams and Dreamtelling: A Group Approach. In J.L. Kleinberg (Ed.), *The Wiley-Blackwell Handbook of Group Psychotherapy* (First Edition, pp. 479–499). Chichester: John Wiley and Sons.

Friedman, R. (2013) Individual or Group Therapy? Indications for Optimal Therapy. *Group Analysis*, 46: 164–170.

Friedman, R. (2014) Group Analysis Today – Developments in Intersubjectivity. *Group Analysis*, 47(3): 194–200.

Loden, S. (2003) The Fate of the Dream in Contemporary Psychoanalysis. *Journal of the American Psychoanalytic Association* (JAPA), 51(1): 43–70.

Mitchell, S.A. (1988) *Relational Concepts in Psychoanalysis.* Cambridge and London: Harvard University Press.

Nitzgen, D. (2010) Hidden Legacies. S.H. Foulkes, Kurt Goldstein and Ernst Cassirer. *Group Analysis*, 43(3): 354–371.

Ogden, T.H. (1996) Reconsidering Three Aspects of Psychoanalytic Technique. *International Journal of Psychoanalysis*, 77(5): 883–900.

Rafaelsen, L. (1996) Projections, Where Do They Go? *Group Analysis*, 29(2): 143–158.

Redl, F. (1942) Group Emotion and Leadership. *Psychiatry*, 5: 573–596.

Segal, H. (1993) The Function of Dreams. In S. Flanders (Ed.), *The Dream Discourse Today* (pp. 100–107). London: Routledge.

Stern, N.D., Sander, L.W., Nahum, P., Harrison, A.M., Lyons-Ruth, K., Morgan, A.C., et al. (1998) Non-Interpretive Mechanisms in Psychoanalytic Therapy: The "Something More" Than Interpretation. *International Journal of Psycho-Analysis*, 79: 903–921.

Ullman, M. (1996) *Appreciating Dreams: A Group Approach.* London: Sage.

Volkan, V.D. (2006) *Killing in the Name of Identity: A Study of Bloody Conflicts.* Charlottesville, VA: Pitchstone Publishing.

Winnicott, D.W. (1965) Ego Distortion in Terms of True and False Self. In *The Maturational Process and the Facilitating Environment: Studies in the Theory of Emotional Development* (pp. 140–152). New York: International UP Inc.

Winnicott, D.W. (1971) *Playing and Reality.* London: Tavistock.

PART II

Who is sick? About pathology in relations

INTRODUCTION TO PART II

Introduction

Relation disorders

Working in group therapy influenced my perspective on pathology. Not too many years after I started to work, I remember sharing with colleagues my feeling that classical individual psychopathology was often not enough to really understand disorders displayed in different situations. Much later, as director of the Technion (Israel's Technical University) Consulting Centre, where every year hundreds of new patients had to be referred to different therapeutic settings, it became clear that psychotherapy lacks a reasonable system of indications. Our indication system is based on sympathy, feelings and hope that the dyadic setting of individual therapy can contain and elaborate almost every problem. There are no clear guidelines about who may be better treated through couple therapy or in a group. My answer to part of this problem was to define Relations Pathology, which is also connected to a setting context.

S.H. Foulkes (1964), who founded group analysis and worked with soldiers' pathology resulting from combat stress, suggested the location of pathology was not in the individual, but in the relations. Following his line of thought 'Relations can make people sick and relations can cure'. Pathology is not only to be found in the individual, but in pathological relations; healthier relations may heal those who could be perceived as dysfunctional people. These perspectives have been corroborated by my experience in group therapy.

Upbringing and education together with 'born' qualities co-create our psyches. But in addition, it is relations and the societal context which may be the big co-creators of a person's pathology (or health). The next chapters contribute to a more relational development of psychoanalytic and group-analytic theory of pathology.

In order to build an indication system, I used Yvonne Agazarian's (1994) research on group developmental phases in order to make a first conceptualization of my four relation disorders. My interpretation of her findings was that fixation to every one of her four stages of group growth development investigated may cause relation pathology. By overcoming fixation, healthier and more efficient functioning could be achieved. I translated her Bionian thinking from a developmental phase to a potential relational pathology, and from the difficulty of an individual, for example the scapegoat, to a reciprocal difficulty in a human connection.

After using my four Disorders as guidelines of an indication system, it became clear that these categories also help to understand the group's dynamic and make more effective interventions. The focus is relation pathology inside the group therapeutic process. Looking at Disorders as a result of a 'failure of containment' of strength/weakness, aggression, pathogenic over-identification or chronic centralization or marginalization provides for new perspectives. All 'partners' in the disordered process are called to participate in an effort to heal difficult emotional problems.

Recently two further developments have built on my four relation disorders. I recommend that this model is used more as an efficient way to describe pathology and contribute to the discovery of more relation disorders. Thus, Yael Doron referred to a romance in the group as a relation disorder and Christoph Seidler added a fifth relation disorder by describing pathology which is caused by relations with authorities. This is the first relation disorder to address specifically pathology in relations with the therapist as leader and an authority.

References

Agazarian, Y. (1994) The Phases of Group Development and the Systems-centred Group. In M. Pines and V. Schermer (Eds.), *Ring of Fire*. London: Routledge.

Foulkes, S.H. (1964) *Therapeutic Group Analysis*. London: Allen and Unwin.

4

WHERE TO LOOK?

Supervising group analysis: A relation disorder perspective[1]

> The primary purpose of supervision is to throw light on the therapeutic relationship; its secondary purpose is to enhance the supervisee skills as a therapist.
>
> *(Behr and Hearst, 2005: 238)*

Without a more sophisticated relations perspective, a therapist cannot facilitate the full potential of the group. Foulkes (1975) thought that the outstanding areas to which interpretations usually refer are the ongoing interactive group processes and the conflict that the individual repeats in the group situation (1975: 124). The therapist who is not aware of the group as a sphere of relational influence may encounter possible difficulties starting from his/her countertransference and the resulting interventions.

Supervision has to promote the therapist's skill in observing relationships – he/she has to learn where to look in the loaded realm of emotions inside the group. Supervising, for me, means to elaborate and help elaborate difficult emotional material, to 'think the thoughts' (Bion, 1992). In other words, the supervisee, the supervisor and the supervision group together create a space that makes everyone's containing abilities available. This partnership works through complex processes. For example, it may use a mental model that is quite structured, one with only certain guidelines or even one totally unstructured. One can describe these models as situated on a continuum, each possessing advantages and disadvantages related to different personalities, stages of professional and individual development, etc. Bion (1970), on the one hand, described a completely open encounter with the patient for a therapist who has 'the capacity to forget, the ability to eschew desire and understanding' (1970: 51) during a psychoanalytic meeting. A non-structured approach may elicit and elaborate emotional processes marginal to consciousness. A more structured approach to supervision may instruct the therapist where to look, what to notice and how to intervene. I believe it is the process of ever-growing integration between structured and non-structured aspects that is helping us improve as therapists. This article presents second thoughts about the guidelines a supervisor may pass on to a group therapist on the issue of pathology and the resulting interventions in group therapy.

Foulkes and his followers worked hard at the translation and transition from individual, dyadic therapy, centring on an intrapsychic view, to the multi-personal, intersubjective space of group analysis. Supervisors and conductors have to deal with both positive and problematic aspects of the psychoanalytic heritage of group analysis.

A relational approach to therapy

The term 'intersubjective' presupposes that the dyad, the smallest group, is indivisible – that we can no longer speak of the patient or the therapist as an isolate. 'Likewise, we cannot speak of the group leader as separate from his group' (Grotstein, 2003: 13). Everyone in close contact participates in the emotional field and will be involved (unconsciously and consciously) in a process of reciprocal influence. It may also mean that an (interpersonal) 'characteristic, like an assumption, will be co-created, maintained and worked through intersubjectively by the linking objects' (Billow, 2003: 40).

Through the inclusion of a relation disorders approach, a new view of pathology may be promoted that enables a more relevant and developed approach to therapy as both personal and interpersonal. One important achievement for the novice group therapist is the development of his/her awareness from a concentration on the individual to that of relations patterns. When the therapist's mind switches to 'object-relating' (Winnicott, 1969), the relevant interventions follow. Object-relating and 'object-use' are the subject matter of group analysis and, although it is accepted in theory, a conductor's automatic reaction will often be to attend to the individual's problems as if he/she were a closed system. The concept of the matrix is based on a consideration of the whole network of communication, using interpersonal 'moments of meeting' (Stern et al., 1998), such as resonance, mirroring and exchange (Zinkin, 1993).

There is a natural tendency for the therapist to 'regress' to treating the private member only. But the therapist's experience is that individual interpretations often remain fruitless if made without an interpersonal context, and usually with good reason: individual changes usually 'surrender' before powerful influences of relations patterns. These interpersonal patterns may be universal, social or cultural givens and sometimes the result of projective identification processes (Rafaelsen, 1996). Either way, it may return us to Freud's (1912) concept of transference as a relational process.

The tendency to look at the individual

Why is this tendency towards addressing the individual pathology so strong? One of the reasons that arises in dialogues with therapists is that the individual is still automatically considered the primary cohesive entity in the group, while 'internal' groups and external relations are more difficult to discern. Moreover, our conservative education at the university teaches us individual nosology (American Psychiatric Association, 1994, *DSM* [*Diagnostic and Statistical Manual*]). As most of the group conductors are also individual therapists, we find that when in stress, the habitual intrapersonal dynamics are easier to detect and address (consciously and unconsciously).

Another reason for addressing individual pathology is that in early childhood we stop blaming others for our sickness and suffering and instead get used to individual medical treatment. Finally, there is a socially embedded unconscious wish to avoid responsibility for the suffering and pathology of others, especially in the social realm. Interestingly, it was Foulkes himself who called our attention to unconscious guilt (and shame?) as a hidden motive for an individual-centered nosology (Foulkes, 1975: 65).

Where to focus?

The fact that it took a long time to accept the existence of transference and to further understand it as an intersubjective relation between container and contained (Bion, 1970) highlights the difficulty of establishing a relational understanding of pathology. Foulkes (1975) tried in principle to develop group analysis as a relationship-centered approach, emphasizing from the beginning, it seems to me, a reciprocal relational perspective when he says, '[Y]ou should *treat the neurotic disturbances, as multipersonal ones*' (1975: 65, my italics), and 'It is not very helpful to speak of individuals in terms of conventional diagnostic labels and to answer the question of indication and counterindication in such terms' (1975: 66).

In contrast to his own therapeutic approach, Foulkes's operational guidelines concentrate more on building a general analytical attitude than on defining focuses of relating and interpreting on the part of the conductor. The analytical attitude concentrates more on 'don'ts' than on 'do's': The conductor's psychological setting should be non-directive, non-manipulative, non-central and he/she should not regard him/herself as the only, or even the most important, transference figure (Foulkes, 1975: 99–155). In this spirit, the conductor should not give 'plunging' interpretations, ever waiting for the group's maturity to show, and many other principles that make analytical group therapy a unique place of secure and steady cure and growth. Analyzing is the main task. Foulkes maintains that 'the analyst's total activity is analyzing . . . the process of establishing and maintaining the group analytic situation . . . the translation of meaning from a less conscious form of communication to a conscious verbal one' (1975: 129). It seems to him '. . . important to analyze . . . and not interpret so fast, as '*interpretation comes in where analysis fails*' (1975: 117, italics in the original text). But where to look when an interpretation is given? Is it the individual or the group-as-a-whole?

The importance of the conductor's focus of attention to the group-analytic process makes re-thinking it imperative. It is difficult to know when to focus on the individual and when to focus on the group. The group-analytic concept of the group as a figure-ground constellation, offering ever-changing configurations of monologue, dialogue and discourse (Schlapobersky, 1993) provides a useful working model and serves as an anchor for trainees who feel themselves tossed from one interaction to another in the group. 'In the end, the trainee usually comes to realize that 'good enough' therapy depends not so much on knowing what is going on, but on being able to hold the setting, providing oneself as a containing presence, facilitating open communication between all in the group (including the conductor) and protecting the group from buffetings which threaten its predictability and safety' (Behr, 1995: 12). We shall now consider that facilitating communication, presence, holding the setting and containing aggression are the conductor's instruments in addition to his/her wish to know 'what is going on', especially in the realm of (pathological) relationships in the group.

Some attempts to define relations pathologies

Focusing on relationships rather than on individual pathology is not new in the young branch of psychotherapy. At the beginning of the last century, Bleuler (1972) describes a pathological relation between humans, 'folie à deux', a contagious craziness that is transmitted within a couple. Recent psychiatric classifications refer to the syndrome as *induced delusional disorder* (DSM-IV) or *shared psychotic disorder* (ICD-10) (American Psychiatric Association, 1994). The slight nuance hints to differences in an interpersonal approach.

Interestingly, only a few other contributions have been made, mainly by those who have had some contact with other than dyadic therapy. Berne (1964) and Minuchin (1974) have made notable contributions.

Bion attempted a differentiation in the process of containment by briefly describing both different qualities of the containing process and varying motivations of the containing partners, naturally resulting in different relationships. By categorizing the container/contained model, Bion (1970) offers a first pathological differentiation attempt. The relationship between container and contained could be either a healthy one (commensual), a regressive-linking one (symbiotic) or a destructive one (parasitic). Billow (2003, 2004) rephrased these three categories of Bion's containment, and translated them into 'symbolic', 'bonding' and 'antilinking'. Commensual is a 'good mother' relation, a reciprocal intersubjective containment partnership, a good enough developed relationship in which *symbolic* activity is reached. In a symbiotic link, a container/contained relationship is prone to a more regressive *bonding*. An (unconscious) *antilinking* connection with a destructive 'parasite' may end in terrorist relating and use of the object (Winnicott, 1969).

'The psychoanalytic problem is the problem of growth and its harmonious resolution in the relationship between the container and the contained repeated in individual, pair and finally group (internal and extra psychically)' (Bion, 1970: 15–16). Rather than a repetition, it seems that in every interpersonal context there is a unique quality of growth to attain. Individuals transit through several settings of relations development: the primal dyad, pair, triangle, small group and large group, all promoting specific qualities of personal and social maturity. Piper and McCallum (1994) have defined five degrees of 'object relations quality', which may be helpful in investigating the growth and development of a relationship. These may also be seen as (non-exhaustive) categories of disorders or degrees of achieved social maturity. Interpersonal maturity may also be relations-dependent as even 'developed' people regress (either manifestly or latently) into exclusively dyadic fantasies and relationships. Later, when acute crises are overcome, more developed relationships can be attained again. Much of the hidden advantages and dynamics of individual therapy is founded in these critical initial aspects, which have to be included in a consideration of indication and selection for group therapy.

Relation disorders – categories

The following is an outline of the pathology of relations that may complement the usual individual approach to mental illness. The concept of containing roles, investigated by Agazarian (1994) is connected to different stages of relations inside groups. It describes primarily the conflict-holder as he/she copes with interpersonal emotional difficulties by 'taking it on him/herself' to elaborate them. I have expanded these descriptions of containing roles to all participants in the group involved in a 'mis-containment' of an emotional difficulty. Relation disorders are mainly the result of such mis-containment.

There are four primal kinds of emotional difficulties that may be ill-contained in society: (1) weakness/strength, (2) aggression, (3) identification/individuation and (4) inclusion/exclusion. Any human being unconsciously 'knows' the experiences of being extremely weak or strong, aggressive and excluded, as exclusive categories of interpersonal pathologies that can only exist as reciprocal complementary emotional movements and as functions of intersubjective processes. As such, the different relation disorders are clustered categories of pathology that differ from the usual individual understanding of illness. They are meant to deepen the group therapist's understanding of therapeutic processes, enabling better treatment through more efficient interventions in group analysis. They may also promote a guide to an optimal selection of the therapeutic environment and a better supervision of group analysis.

1. Deficiency relation disorders

This is a relationship in which strong and weak individuals in reciprocal communication compulsively use subjective illness and suffering. The powerful and the disempowered interact in groups or subgroups around dreaded suffering. Latent and manifest communication maintains a split as a result of the difficulties in containing deficiency and strength. As a result, weaknesses and power are projected into partial object relations, resulting in relations between those who seem extremely weak and those who are felt to be very powerful. In this disorder, (unconscious) guilt towards the distressed seems to play an *including* role. On the one hand, it promotes help; on the other, it continuously reinforces the split positions, establishing relationships based on sickness and weakness instead of health and strength. A related interpersonal pathology, usually reflecting the suffering side of the deficiency relation disorders, is called 'The Identified Patient' (Minuchin, 1974). It is used for the sick member of family relationships, who is believed to reciprocally contribute to the creation of various mental diseases through projecting and identifying mechanisms. The deficiency relation disorders describes a more general interpersonal difficulty to contain weakness, distress and childish dependency or/and strength. It establishes two spaces-in-relation: one which cannot feel safety if it feels weakness, and has to project it, and another which learns not to feel safety without exhibiting deficiencies and projecting power on to others.

2. Rejection relation disorders

Failing to contain aggression may result in the creation of a scapegoating environment. This shared illness is based both consciously and unconsciously on strong hostilities, which are acted out towards deviant and usually weak members of society. Pathological interactions like displaced hate, violent rejection and expulsion create a community atmosphere that pushes to the exclusion of the distressed. A group's illusionary safe space is achieved by denying the rejected a safe space (Friedman, 2004, 2006; Kotani, 2004) after the rejection of the needy and weak members fuels a remorseless aggressive expulsion. In this disorder (unconscious) guilt towards the distressed seems to play an *excluding* role.

3. Selfless relation disorders

A society in need of a sacrifice will coerce a devoted member, who usually has failed to contain separation, to engage in selfless behaviour. The results of this over-identification may be heroism or self-mutilation. The use of power and education, selfishly abusing others by promoting selflessness, colludes with social and individual inability to contain processes of separation and autonomy. If the individual self does not have his/her own safe space in which to develop, the result may be both the physical and psychical martyrdom of the individual, encouraged by an idealizing or abusing society. The community will be endangered by harmful patterns, including tendencies toward dependency and excessive use of violence.

4. Exclusion relation disorders

The more a community copes with social failure and disappointment through splitting, projection and evacuation, the more it will exclude marginal members and create 'outsiders'. The inability to contain socially less able and disempowered members means that individuals and subgroups will be marginalized. The secure centre of society will be the realm of the majority, but many will undergo an isolation process, which will tend to become chronic. In this relation disorder, a safe space is established for members who belong to the (sometimes small) majority or to the 'norm' by distancing others. It is not an active rejection that characterizes this disorder, but rather the exclusion of 'outsiders'. The reciprocal relation between the excluders and the socially weak will maintain itself by intersubjective processes, and will lead to unproductiveness, suffering of the marginalized members and the activation of powerful passive-aggressive components. Many of our patients seem to suffer inside this relation disorder.

Relation disorders and supervision

Every disorder is the result of reciprocal interactions of all participants, including the conductor. In a small group it may be enough that one participant does not participate in the pathological interaction to disable the pathological interaction. In each relation disorder the conductor's (unconscious) interaction with the 'containing role' and the group may be of interest with regard to the supervision process. Because of the intersubjective influence of all participants, including the conductor, the latter has the potential possibility to promote or treat the relation disorder. In the case of the Deficiency Disorder, it is clear that the conductor is easily seduced, because of his/her professional tendency to 'treat' the weak and sick and unconsciously promote a strong/weak relationship through therapeutic interactions. In the rejection relation disorders, the supervisor has to help focus on the interaction that promotes a displacement of aggression towards a scapegoat. The 'heroes' of the selfless relation disorders evoke in others reinforcing behaviour that promotes an ever-stronger social role-suction for the heroes. As a result there is an over-identification that makes it more difficult to separate from a selfless life. Another much experienced example of the difficulties encountered with Exclusion Disorders is that the conductor represses his/her contribution to the marginalization of a participant or his/her subgroup. In spite of his/her wish not to harm anyone, there may be an Oedipal move towards the marginalization of others, which allows the central participants (again, including the group therapist) to enjoy societal status more than ever. Supervision may often be the only place where it is possible to work through the unconscious motivations that help establish and maintain a relation disorder.

Examples

An awareness and deep understanding of the existence of an interpersonal pathology may create relational interventions. The therapist must be able to address intersubjective patterns, which are neither necessarily group-as-a-whole nor individual. Focusing on relations complements the group-analytic exchange between a particular participant and the group, implying that subgroups may be carriers and loci of pathology. Heightening awareness of relation disorders also contributes to the creation of possible ways to change the pattern. Practising to focus on relations may be difficult without the support of supervision.

There is no group I know of that does not have an example of the deficiency relation disorders. Every community has within it a relationship that enacts the feeling that someone is flawed and inferior, while some respond to the need to be strong and superior by caring for the weak and needy. If this becomes compulsive, the group is 'using' the relationship to split emotional difficulties. The group's persistent positive response to the individual's obsessive manifestation of weakness and deficiency promotes a pathological relational pattern. The reciprocal relationship between weakness and sickness on the one hand and strength and health on the other is fascinatingly complex. Often a group is healthy enough to refuse invasion of its space by a new member's feelings of anxiety, depression, etc. But a group may start to collaborate willingly with obsessive inferiority and worthlessness, sometimes as a result of guilt or other empathic feelings. Meanwhile, the emotional atmosphere becomes unbearable for some members, who cope with this stress by massive splitting of deficiency feelings. These feelings are projected onto the weak member, who, used to identifying with the projected weakness, seems ever more needy and suffering: in order for the group members to find safety from weakness, it is projected and placed on to someone who is used to feeling safe only if he/she feels weak.

It is usually more helpful to approach this kind of pattern from the relations perspective rather than from the personal. The social gains of being in an interaction with the group are much stronger than any personal motivation to end the suffering. People are entirely social beings and the primal need to relate is not to be put at risk. The possibility of relating differently evokes insecurity regarding one's capabilities of attachment through a different role. To be capable or experienced in another approach may evoke dreadful anxieties. Conversely, the possibility of getting 'good feelings' from an interaction with a needy person, whilst distancing weakness and anxieties, is unconsciously more rewarding than any change into healthy relationships. A therapeutic relational approach challenges the unconscious, mutual agreement between the deficient and the healthy. Interpreting the general disavowal of dreadful weakness should go together with addressing the deviant individual's constant willingness to act as the patient.

Vignettes

An analytic group started to empathize strongly with a very depressed woman immediately after her joining the group. This pattern increased in strength over several months – the depressive participant had already gone through many years of role-reinforcement inside and outside individual therapy. It was by using the discomfort of some group members regarding the weakness and the need to comfort her that a different relationship was made possible between her and the group, enabling both sides to become aware of the gains.

A relationship in a group around a 'scapegoat' is a good example of the rejection relation disorders.

> After M had been idealized for a while, the group started becoming increasingly more disappointed in him. A young, professionally successful man, he

> had, until that point, been considered quite an interesting person. The longer this process of disappointment went on, the stronger the emotions it evoked. A subgroup felt that M was only playing with the group and his false self seemed to awaken its every resistance. He could not be trusted, they said, and one could not be sure if he used his impressive abilities for or against you. This group already tended to discharge strong tensions in violent ways, encountering difficulties in containing much of the turmoil intrinsic to emotional relationships. Maybe because he had been a much admired participant, a large part of the group now felt an even stronger urge to expel the 'fake'. It was as if they hated this person, who reacted to the rejection and isolation with strong needs to be loved and accepted. These needs, in turn, were felt to be a fake, untrustworthy move, which strengthened the rejection. At a certain moment, it seemed as if a safe space could only be established by displacing anger into aggressive acting out on to this scapegoat, who usually treated himself as completely impotent.

In supervision, possible countertransference reactions were suggested, since it was possible that the conductor was using the scapegoating process to defend himself against becoming the target of aggression.

Differing from individual therapy, where threatening aggression is often displaced from the therapist against outsiders, parents etc., in groups it is displaced to weaker participants. The distinct place of the group conductor makes him/her an important participant in the development of the rejection relation disorders as one who sometimes profits from the resulting destructive interactions. Interpreting individual latent motivations here was also felt to be less efficient than a relational approach to the rejection displayed: all of the participants in the relationship tried to work on their awareness and change their containing. Reciprocal work on violent tendencies in the group and many of the participants' difficulties in containing tensions, fears and the resulting transformation into aggression went together with the investigation of the scapegoat's own contribution to being the recipient of the group's rejection. In this group, work was done on the defensive purpose of displacement of interpersonal aggression and the resulting destructive interactions.

The selfless disorder

There are gender differences in all relation disorders, but this is especially true in the Selfless Disorder. Women and men usually exhibit a great diversity of behaviour regarding selflessness, although for both genders it can be subsumed in putting oneself at the service of others. For women, however, this is seen as doing 'good' while for men it is seen as more destructive behaviour, sometimes even as doing 'bad'. The selfless 'bitch', described elsewhere (Friedman, 2005), is an exemplification of this third relation disorder – a relationship between a subgroup of needy participants and a woman who only wanted to 'do good' for others. The pathology lies in the compulsive repetition of the reciprocal pattern. The woman does not have the choice of drawing the group's attention to her own suffering self and the others do not feel the need to give her something significant. The group was using her, and she was eager to be 'used'. Both selfishness and selflessness exhibit themselves primarily as ego-syntonic feelings. Shared by the participants of the relation disorder, it may be understood as an (over)identification with the pattern of dedication and taking. This woman used to behave in the group as she behaved in reality – as if everyone were her concern and on her mind. She would be interested in what happened between sessions, would give advice and would easily give up her own work for the 'benefit of others'. She was a caring person, and did not even usually feel neglected, since a lot of needy people asked for her energy and attention. However, the fact that she had been married many times and felt deeply dissatisfied with her 'husbands' attitudes' towards her were early signs. The group was using her and she 'agreed' to be used in a form of relating that was not given to choice.

Two elements, both interpersonal, seem to have been crucial in the subsequent development. First, it was important that she and the group started to openly accept selfish behaviour, which became both legitimate and open to scrutiny in the matrix. This helped her to make selfishness a learned skill and an increasingly possible behavioural choice.

Thus, disorders cure each other.

The other transformative element was the attacks she received while trying to be selfless. It was at this point that the group's resistance to feeling 'serviced' by her, while feelings of being patronized created an angry outburst in which the expression 'selfless bitch' was coined.

The conductor had to work repeatedly on his (conscious) sympathies and unconscious identifications with the selfless role in order to influence the relational disorder in another direction.

Curing and developing through all relation disorders

In the four years N was in an analytic group, he went through all of the disorders. When he finally ended in the exclusion relation disorders, he felt he had made the greatest progress of his life. In the 15 years of his previous individual therapy, he had been treated as having a paranoid character disorder. Married for the second time, he encountered many problems in his parenting of the two children from both marriages. He felt and exhibited strong spells of envy. This was also the case at work, a very high-powered enterprise, where he provoked periodic conflicts stimulated by his jealous attitude and his fears of being rejected. He felt very frustrated in all his close connections by his suspicions of exclusion and rejection. The smallest frustrating interpersonal interaction, whether with his wife, his children or his colleagues, would ignite an openly angry outburst followed by depressive narcissistic injury.

In the first two years of his analytic group treatment, he often felt unwanted, rejected and that all his efforts to build a safe space were shattered (Friedman, 2004). In the first year and half the main effort was to 'treat' N in the 'conventional' way, which he at times dedicated himself to with the considerable abilities for intrapsychic scrutiny that he had learned in his years in individual therapy. The conductor had the feeling all the while that working through his envy and jealousy mechanisms, as well as others, was fruitless. The group (including the conductor) collaborated with N in centring him as the crazy participant (which he was, in a way). His suspicious spells were analysed and for a short time, the threat of the whole group's disappointment and rage dissipated in the split reciprocal attitude. N also was suspicious, but made an effort to trust and contain his hate. The main dynamic issue for the group at this stage was keeping the matrix from having a weak/strong split between normal/crazy protagonists. It needed much supervision in order not to over-concentrate on the therapy of this patient.

Soon the group also felt hurt and attacked. Some participants starting to take revenge through scorn and counter-attacks, and others joined in what seemed to be a move towards excluding N from the group. N periodically fell into spells of passive-aggressive reciprocation during these two years or so. It seemed a great insight and relief when he openly admitted that he also became envious and suspicious whenever his wife 'invested' more in his son than in him.

Apparently, more significant change happened through interpersonal efforts than through intrapsychic interpretations. A deeper analytical understanding was promoted in all group members, but proved ineffective in changing attitudes and relationships. N's efforts to contain the suspicion and cope with his rage and hatred helped him and the group get out of a compulsive conflictual and paranoid atmosphere, which contaminated every encounter. For the first time in his life, he was able to comply with the group's culture while experiencing less destructive rivalry and antagonism. The group had been quite experienced and mature in its responses from the beginning, and exhibited a keen ability to interpret and reframe his attacks on linking.

Containing capacities of groups vary and may depend on their experience or member composition. This specific group may also have been affected by the fact that N had joined the group around the same time as D, which seems to have fostered a special bond between them. This relationship was also a kind of special source of support and security for N, although it was not excluded from tension. The supervision helped the conductor work with both N and the other group members. Significant emotional movement began in the relationship with the outside world when his incredulity of the group's intention towards him, as well as the group's hidden emotional response of angry hurt and withdrawal, were repeatedly and openly addressed. In the end, a greater group ability to contain both N's and its own rage and conflicting emotions was achieved.

However, this was not achieved until developments, in the course of struggling with two different relation disorders, were overcome: first, the relationship between his role as the group's selfless worker and the group, and finally, his being stranded in a marginalized position. Every group has 'heroes' that are a configuration of their environment. Selflessness has both universal and culturally specific characteristics. In therapy groups, a relationship may revolve around an insightful hero. He may be (mis-)used by the group as the one who is completely open. Almost every emotion goes through him, he does not refuse any suggestions and the group continuously reinforces his over-identification with the togetherness. His wish for acceptance was so great, and his over-identification so pervasive, that for a while a relationship is established between a (pseudo-)container for everything, one who has to take everything in and share it boundlessly, and the group, who can evacuate into the container at will. This relationship is not really interdependent, but is rather a completely dependent relationship, a symbiotic containment in which identification with the perpetrator is complete and has even destructive antilinking characteristics. For a significant period of some months, the connections in the group surrounding N had this psychological heroic quality – while being satisfying for most of them only after interpreting several aspects of the relationship did its pathological character became clear. Mostly by helping all members concerned verbalize aspects of (what was later felt as) the great taboo of paranoia – the partly right and partly wrong perception of being rejected and hurt by the group – as well as retaliation fantasies, a significant drop in tension could be achieved.

The group's openness about feelings seemed to help N not feel 'crazy in his mind' on the one hand, and on the other, facilitated the members' experience of the reciprocal influence of hurt, envy, hate, rejection and eventual (mostly passive) aggression. The reciprocal openness helped the process of 'ego training in action' (Foulkes, 1964: 82): exercising and bearing (tolerating) the group's resonance to the suspicious interactions, and working them by mirroring. His final position as a somewhat marginal but not rejected member of society, a sometimes frustrated but relatively contained and containing human being, who does not have to act out, is an interesting point in the 'depressive position' (Klein, 1935, 1960). It means that perhaps we attained the limit of health he could bear.

In 1946, Major Foulkes (as he then was) wrote: 'The therapist . . . knew that, while digging a tunnel from one end, he would be met halfway by workers from the other end' (1946: 86).

Note

This paper is based on lectures given at the EGATIN conference in Split, Croatia (June 2004), the Israel Institute of Group Analysis and the Israel Conference on Group Supervision.

1 This chapter appeared previously as Friedman, R. (2007) Where to Look? Supervising Group Analysis – A Relations Disorder Perspective. *Group Analysis*, Vol. 40(2):251–268, Sage.

References

Agazarian, Y.M. (1994) The Phases of Group Development and the Systems-centered Group. In V.L. Shermer and M. Pines (Eds.), *Ring of Fire* (pp. 36–86). London: Routledge.

American Psychiatric Association (1994) *Diagnostic and Statistical Manual and Mental Disorders* (Fourth Edition). Washington, DC: American Psychiatric Association.

Behr, H. (1995) The Integration Between Theory and Practice. In M. Sharpe (Ed.), *The Third Eye: Supervision of Analytic Groups* (pp. 4–17). London: Routledge.

Behr, H. and Hearst, L. (2005) *Group Analytic Psychotherapy: A Meeting of Minds*. London and Philadelphia, PA: Whurr.

Berne, E. (1964) *Games People Play*. New York: Random House.

Billow, R.M. (2003) *Relational Group Psychotherapy: From Basic Assumptions to Passion*. London: Jessica Kingsley.

Billow, R.M. (2004) Working Relationally With the Adolescent in Group. *Group Analysis*, 37(2): 187–200.

Bion, W.R. (1970) *Attention and Interpretation*. London: Heinemann. Reprinted in *Seven Servants: Four Works by Wilfred R. Bion*. New York: Aronson, 1977.

Bion, W.R. (1992) *Cogitations*. London: Karnac.

Bleuler, E. (1972) *Lehrbuch der Psychiatrie*. Heidelberg: Springer.

Foulkes, S.H. (1946, May) Principles and Practice of Group Therapy, by Major S.H. Foulkes. *R.A.M.C. (Royal Army Medical Corps)*, 10: 85–89.

Foulkes, S.H. (1964) *Therapeutic Group Analysis*. London: Maresfield Library.

Foulkes, S.H. (1975) *Group Analytic Psychotherapy, Method and Principle*. London and New York: Karnac.

Freud, S. (1912) *The Dynamics of Transference* (Standard Edition, Vol. 12). London: Hogarth Press, 1958.

Friedman, R. (2004) Safe Space and Relational Pathology. *International Journal of Counseling and Psychotherapy*, 2: 108–114.

Friedman, R. (2005) *Disorders Heal Each Other in Group Analysis – A Relational Perspective*, Unpublished Paper for the Israel Institute for Group Analysis.

Friedman, R. (2006) Who Contains the Group and Who Is the Leader? A Relational Disorders Perspective. *European Journal of Psychotherapy & Counselling*, 8(1): 21–32.

Grotstein, J.S. (2003) Introduction. In R.M. Billow (Ed.), *Relational Group Psychotherapy: From Basic Assumptions to Passion*. London: Jessica Kingsley.

Klein, M. (1935) Contribution to the Psychogenesis of Manic-Depressive States. In *Developments in Psycho-Analysis*. London: Hogarth, 1948.

Klein, M. (1960) Symposium on 'Depressive Illness' – A Note on Depression in the Schizophrenic. *International Journal of Psycho-Analysis*, 41: 509–511.

Kotani, H. (2004) Safe Space in a Psychodynamic World. *International Journal of Counseling and Psychotherapy*, 2: 87–92.

Minuchin, S. (1974) *Families and Family Therapy*. Boston, MA: Harvard University Press.

Piper, M. and McCallum, M. (1994) Selection of Patients for Group Interventions. In H.S. Bernard and P. MacKenzie (Eds.), *Basics of Group Psychotherapy*. New York and London: Guilford Press.

Rafaelsen, L. (1996) Projections, Where Do They Go? (19th S.H. Foulkes Lecture). *Group Analysis*, 29(2): 143–158.

Schlapobersky, J. (1993) The Language of the Group: Monologue, Dialogue and Discourse in Group Analysis. In D. Brown and L. Zinkin (Eds.), *The Psyche and the Social World: Developments in Group-Analytic Theory* (pp. 211–231). London: Routledge.

Stern, D., Sandler, L., Nahum, J., Harrison, A., Lyons-Ruth, K., Morgan, A., Bruschweiler-Stern, N. and Tronick, E. (1998) Non-Interpretative Mechanisms in Psychoanalytic Therapy. *International Journal of Psycho-Analysis*, 79: 903–921.

Winnicott, D.W. (1969) The Use of an Object and Relating Through Identifications. In *Playing and Reality*. London: Tavistock, 1971.

Zinkin, L. (1993) Exchange as a Therapeutic Factor in Group Analysis. In D. Brown and L. Zinkin (Eds.), *The Psyche and the Social World: Developments in Group Analytic Theory* (pp. 99–117). London: Routledge.

5

INDIVIDUAL OR GROUP THERAPY?

Indications for optimal therapy[1]

Why group therapy?

Group therapists often feel very clear about the advantages of their particular approach. Yet it is not always easy to convey the unique benefits that come from participation in groups, especially median groups. Having a clearer indication for different spaces of treatment (individual, groups, couples and family therapy) could help to define the unique contribution of small and median groups.

Example

Uri was 40, married with three children, felt internally insecure, anxious and particularly tense whenever he had to meet in a group. These symptoms did not change in spite of two 'satisfactory' individual therapies – and in great contrast to his professional success and his social life.

Group therapy, indications and optimal treatment

What makes small and median group therapy unique enough to justify a clear indication? How shall therapists be convinced that participation in group therapy is absolutely imperative? We are in need of a good enough indication system, which connects specific disorders with specific treatment strategies. Acute knee pain can be screened and diagnosed so that you know if and when you need either rest for your knee, physiotherapy or an operation. The physician's suggestions may not be ego-syntonic or understandable to every patient. Nonetheless, patients tend to follow an indication for their optimal therapy.

Similarly, in psychotherapy we should ask: *What* is the disorder that needs to be treated? *What* is the *optimal* therapeutic *space*, and *when* should a specific optimal *space* be recommended?

1. *What* disorder should be treated?

Should disorders to be treated only be defined in terms of the individual? Or perhaps they should be defined interpersonally? Classical individual pathologies such as depression or OCD reflect of course the traditional and common approach, although they often are not specific enough to serve as a particular indication for therapy. A narcissistic disorder can feel acceptable in a personal relationship but not in the family network, or vice versa. And it may not feel acceptable in a group. Other perspectives for optimal therapy may be found in approaches such as psychological mindedness (McCallum and Piper, 1990) or object quality of relations (McCallum et al., 2003)[2] In these approaches personal abilities in internal and external relations have been specified and their indication for group therapy have been investigated. I want to suggest another possibility, namely, defining disorders, which are specifically *interpersonal* and *multi-personal.* This will serve the psychotherapist in differentiating between groups, couples, families and individual therapy spaces – and which of these are appropriate treatment modalities for particular disorders.

Example

Uri was diagnosed as having experienced traumatic ostracism as a teenager, which led to great isolation and hurt. In spite of subsequent, good social development, a sense of basic insecurity remained when engaging with groups, and he needed to periodically retreat into dyadic protection.

Defining relation disorders: a fundamental turn of mind

In the evolution of the depth psychologies, psychoanalysis developed in a manner consonant with Freud's early premises as they presented themselves in classical individual theory. Then, Fairbairn and Balint, the former in Scotland and the latter in Hungary, working from very different starting points, each took the presenting detail of neurotic psychopathology and, in the 1930s, offered clinicians *a fundamental turn of mind.* They suggested that behind the symptomatic picture lay a basic relational problem at the pre-Oedipal level. According to Fairbairn, most neurotic symptoms reflected unresolved dependency needs and, according to Balint, a faulty attachment pattern that he called 'the basic fault'. Out of their fundamental turn of mind, object relations theory was created.

A generation later in the 1950s, Nathan Ackerman, Lyman Wynne and other early family therapists took issue with the existing view of the individual as the 'unit' of psychopathology and introduced another *fundamental turn of mind* by citing the attachment itself – the relational bond – as the issue for investigation and therapy. Foulkes worked under the impulse of this same trajectory of revision to bring transpersonal phenomena to the foreground.

I suggest here that it is now possible to propose categories of relational disorder for which group therapy is uniquely suited as the therapy of choice. In order to introduce the concept of relation disorders, we do well to cite Foulkes (1975: 66) 'It is not very helpful to speak of individuals in terms of conventional diagnostic labels'. And further: we '. . . should *treat the "neurotic disturbance, as multipersonal ones"*' (Foulkes, 1975: 65, my italics)'. '[T]ranspersonal phenomena goes to the very roots of any approach to group psychology and requires a *fundamental turn of mind*' (Foulkes, 1964: 18). I suggest here a contemporary *fundamental turn of mind* by adding relation disorders to our classic definition for individual pathology. Using the complementary optic of multi-personal dysfunctions will not only improve indications for psychotherapy but also facilitate optimal contribution of the different therapeutic spaces;[3] e.g. most of the following relation disorders may not even appear in the dyadic therapeutic space.

Relation disorders are multi-personal dysfunctional patterns (Friedman, 2005, 2006 and 2007). They are categories of reciprocal emotional and behaviour patterns detectable in society and group therapy. These disorders are co-created, interpersonal dysfunctions patterns, which are the result of a failure of all involved parties, e.g., failure to contain strong emotions, such as separation anxieties and needs for inclusion and aggression. The following are preliminary descriptions of interpersonal dysfunctions, categories of disorders based on Agazarian's research of group functioning (Agazarian, 1994).

A. In the *deficiency relation disorder* there is an inability of the participants to contain the duality between weakness and strength in oneself and others. A group participant or a subgroup will feel chronically deficient, communicating anxious, depressive and inferiority messages in the interaction with others who are fixated by feelings of being functional, powerful and helpful. The split between what is called in family therapy 'the Identified Patient' and its counterpart: 'the Identified Caretaker' will often immobilize a group's relations and create chronic pathology.

B. The *rejection*[4] *relation disorder* results from an inability to contain the group's aggression. Increasingly strong fantasized violence between a rejecting subgroup and an inclusion-starved individual may be acted out. Additional processes such as the tendency to scapegoat without guilt and shame on the one hand and the scapegoat's increasing neediness to be included becomes surprisingly strong. The complementary relationship between rejected and rejecters in school classes and closed societies are pathogenic in more ways than one. These tendencies increase as modern communication makes it possible to reject facelessness.

C. By *relation disorders of the self* a pathological relationship is specified, in which social over-identification results in an under-development of an autonomic, mature Self. Selfless 'heroes' (Agazarian, 1994) and their 'selfish' counterparts collude (in a gender-wise, different way) to serve the 'cause' while harming themselves and others. While women and men are educated to selflessly offer their lives for their families, communities and jobs, they become obsessively preoccupied with the sense of heroic using, and being misused by society, while also using and misusing others at the same time. This under-development affects the genders differently in contents, while presenting similar processes of harm to the Self.

D. In the *exclusion relation disorder*, the core of a society does not wish to destroy individuals or subgroups but nonetheless acts to marginalize them. This phenomenon becomes a chronic illness for a group or society when the excluded accept marginalization, and no movement between the centre and margins is possible. Symptoms, which resemble a depression or an OCD may develop, resulting in a generally less than optimal level of energy, productivity and satisfaction in the whole group. Different ethnic groups, as well as 'different' people, such as women (still), homosexuals, ex-convicts, the poor and black, the ex-psychotic and many other communities are included in chronic marginalization. Good enough psychic adjustments must include membership in small groups that move from the margins to the centre and back again and can create a significant output. All forms of dysfunctional relations with the centre may be transformed in small, median or large groups (de Maré, 2002; Pisani, 2000). Only mutual changes of all involved will result in a movement to health.

Example

Uri went through group analysis, in which he worked mainly on three dysfunctional patterns consecutively:

His panic about becoming a scapegoat was elaborated in the relations between him and the group.

1 Mutual tendencies to avoid and reject along with a longing for irrational inclusion were worked through.
2 Later, the ambivalence about being a 'weak' person and maintaining a strong facade in the group were elaborated in connection with deficient relation disorders.

The characteristic pathological interactions were uniquely re-enacted in the group where they could eventually be appropriately treated, promoting a better circumscribed Indication. Eventually, Uri and the group succeeded in enlarging their freedom to choose a 'hero', or to selflessly give some of their own space away.

2. *What* is the *optimal* therapeutic *space*?

For many reasons, *relation disorders, characterized by dysfunctional patterns, need to be treated where they were created.* In group analysis, the human need to re-enact patterns is treated through 'ego training in action' (Foulkes, 1968: 181). Differentiating between the *presence* of a dysfunctional pattern and the *therapeutic value* of a specific space helps us to answer the question: When is the median group indicated as optimal treatment for relation disorders?

From my clinical experience I would say that at least three relation disorders (the 2nd, 3rd, 4th) will be uniquely (re-)enacted in small and median groups. Because of the need to intervene with all the sides that *reciprocally* contribute to conflict, median groups will be most efficient in the elaboration of the 3rd and 4th relation disorder (small groups probably more on the 1st and 2nd RDs). The possibility of elaboration will vary according to the intensity of the affects, e.g., hate, envy. The measure of destructive feelings and motivation or amount of emotional dysfunction will influence the optimal size of a working group for the treatment of relation disorders.

In Israel we have learned that for the treatment of social traumata, median group is clearly the optimal curing space. Experiences after the Second Lebanese War, when the North of Israel was in the process of recovering from the traumatic impact of thousands of rockets, have demonstrated that median groups were particularly efficient in working through feelings of exclusion, helplessness and defensive over-identification.

3. *When* will a specific optimal *space* be recommended?

Most potential patients prefer to start with individual therapy.[5] Newcomers to therapy are rather vulnerable and fear what they imagine will be group non-containment and lack of protection. When we feel acutely bad, we automatically shout: 'Mamma' and not: 'Parents' or 'Family'! The longing for care, soothing and protection in dyadic-kinds of therapy are connected with emotional experiences in the early mother-child relationship. Thus, rather than weigh a deeper or more specific Indication that would include median or small group therapy, we habitually turn to the unconscious promise of the individual therapy setting. I am suggesting, in a fundamental turn of mind, that we begin to adopt a two-step indications approach. This means that we should accept that the majority of patients will start therapy in the dyadic space. However, soon afterward, it would be wise for therapist and patient to consider group therapy as a next optimal treatment step. To bring about change in multi-personal dysfunctions, the group therapy space offers optimal possibilities.

Notes

1 This chapter appeared previously as Friedman, R (2013) Individual or Group Therapy? Indications for Optimal Therapy. *Group Analysis*, 46: 164–170.
2 PM is defined as the ability to identify conflictual dynamic components, e.g., wishes, anxiety, defences, and to relate them to a person's difficulties. OQR is defined as a person's tendency to establish certain kinds of relationships with others. It refers to the quality of a person's lifelong pattern of relationships, not just current or recent relationships. Interviewers assess a contender for therapy by looking at five levels of relationships: mature, triangular, controlling, searching and primitive.
3 In addition to intervening into processes on the 'group-as-a-whole' or on individual levels, this perspective may also sharpen our vision on specific relationship categories.
4 I define rejection as more aggressive and qualitatively different than exclusion. Rejection means pushing out of the group, while exclusion means pushing towards the group's margins.
5 Some, who are afraid of intimacy, avoid requesting (individual) therapy.

References

Agazarian, Y.M. (1994) The Phases of Group Development and the Systems-Centered Group. In V.L. Schermer and M. Pines (Eds.), *Ring of Fire: Primitive Affects and Object Relations in Group Psychotherapy* (pp. 36–86). London: Routledge.

de Maré, P. (2002) The Millennium and the Median Group. *Group Analysis*, 35(2): 195–208.

Foulkes, S.H. (1964) *Therapeutic Group Analysis*. London: George Allen and Unwin.

Foulkes, S.H. (1968) Group Dynamic Processes and Group Analysis. In E. Foulkes (Ed.), *Selected Papers* (pp. 175–186). London: Karnac.

Foulkes, S.H. (1975) *Group-Analytic Psychotherapy: Method and Principles*. London: Gordon and Breach. Reprinted London: Karnac, 1986.

Friedman, R. (2005) *Disorders Heal Each Other in Group Analysis – A Relation Pathology Perspective*. www.funzionegamma.edu

Friedman, R. (2006) Who Contains the Group and Who Is the Leader? *European Journal of Psychotherapy and Counselling*, 8(1): 21–32.

Friedman, R. (2007) Where to Look? Supervising Group Analysis – A Relation Disorder Perspective. *Group Analysis*, 40(2): 251–268.

McCallum, M. and Piper, W.E. (1990) The Psychological Mindedness Assessment Procedure. *Psychological Assessment*, 2: 412–418.

McCallum, M., Piper, W.E., Ogrodniczuk, J.S. and Joyce, W.E. (2003) Relationships Among Psychological Mindedness, Alexithymia and Outcome in Four Forms of Short-term Psychotherapy. *Psychology and Psychotherapy*, 76: 133–144.

Pisani, R. (2000) The Median Group in Clinical Practice: An Experience of Eight Years. *Group Analysis*, 33(1): 77–90.

6

GROUP ANALYSIS TODAY

Developments in intersubjectivity[1]

Introduction

The intersubjective perspective of human relatedness implies a permeability of the psyche together with a reciprocal influence. This differentiates group analysis from many other approaches. Foulkes, who certainly was a pioneer in the understanding of the interpersonal dimension, took Freud's meeting of the unconscious, which in many ways was marginalized for decades in psychoanalysis, one step further. Freud wrote:

> To put it in a formula: [the analyst] must turn his own unconscious like a receptive organ towards the transmitting unconscious of the patient. He must adjust himself to the patient as a telephone receiver is adjusted to the transmitting microphone. Just as the receiver converts back into soundwaves the electric oscillations in the telephone line which were set up by sound waves, so the doctor's unconscious is able, from the derivatives of the unconscious which are communicated to him, to reconstruct that unconscious, which has determined the patient's free associations.
>
> *(1912: 115)*

Already in 1948 Foulkes defines an unconscious, primordial connection between group participants as *transpersonal*. By this concept he means that people in the matrix are intersubjectively connected 'as if X-rays would pass between them' (Foulkes, 1948: 1). Based on this view of the Matrix, Foulkes describes a space built on human interconnectivity in which different communications, introjections and projections and other elements build a network. There, influential stimuli co-create relations embedded in multilayer communication.

In the absence of a better explanation as to how this *transpersonality* functions, it is possible to adopt the concept of projective identification, contagion (Redl,

1942) and other connecting devices. Projective identification is a Kleinian concept which tries to describe the reciprocal emotional elaboration between container and contained and is described by Rafaelson, in a Foulkes lecture, as the most important communicative mechanism in the matrix (Rafaelson, 1996).

Recognizing the similarity between the transpersonal concept and intersubjective approaches confronts us with some technical dilemmas. The modern relational approach (Mitchell, 1988) raises questions about neutrality and other related areas – especially the way in which intersubjectivists use this reciprocal permeability in our close therapeutic relations, e.g. the analyst's need for more transparency in the group may be something some of the group-analytic conductors may find difficult to agree with. I have found that even some of the clinical and theoretical implications of the transpersonal approach to dreams, communication and phantasy may be difficult to be digested and accepted by conductors.

For example, my findings that dreaming may be a mechanism used not only by our own Self, but by others, including the group, may be difficult to accept. Indeed the transpersonal/intersubjective perspectives suggest that the borders between our Psyches are more permeable than we often like to think (Friedman, 2012). Social Dreaming (Lawrence, 2007) may be a perfect example of the manifestation of intersubjectivity in the group as-a-whole. While being a method for identifying cultural knowledge and a way of finding 'the social truth' through dream representation, all informational processes may be influential and transformational of society.

In fact, understanding the relatedness with other individuals, groups and society may be crucial for the future of our trade, and an appreciation of the intersubjective helps us to rethink these concepts. Weegmann (2011) and Lavie (2011) raise questions about possible changes in the practice of group analysis as a result of the intersubjective perspective.

Making space for the appreciation of both sympathy and empathy in the study of human relations, Husserl (1931) introduces his concept of intersubjectivity within the context of a general discussion of phenomenology. The intersubjective concept has enabled a more complete conceptualization of the relationship experience by humans who are both subjects and objects of this experience. Moreover, from this perspective the experience of oneself is defined in terms of how one has been experienced by another in terms of this shared internal world of relations.

The recognition of intersubjectivity has created a new psychological paradigm in which the individual is regarded by definition a 'person-in-relation' (e.g. Hopper, 2003; Grotstein, 2002). Although the famous dictum that 'there is no such thing as a baby' (Winnicott, 1958) refers to the fact that in the beginning of life the newborn is totally dependent on his mother, this statement has come to be a metaphor for the social-psychological interdependence and inter-relation of mother and child throughout infancy and childhood at least. Intersubjectivity implies reciprocal relations in which both sides have a great impact on the other, and neither is found to be a neutral, not important player. Even a baby is not a passive being, unilaterally controlled by his genetic, instinctual or his experiential fate alone, but a 'competent new born' (Friedman and Vietze, 1972). This active baby both co-creates his human environment, and is reciprocally co-dependent on mutual responses from and with other subjects.

These two intersubjective aspects reflect a central paradoxical perspective of human existence: on the one hand, the sometimes painful individual's dependency on society and his mind's permeability to external influences and, on the other hand, the individual's potential power over others and his ability to co-create relational situations show different perspectives of the intersubjective side of relationship.

The term 'intersubjective' presupposes that the classical therapeutic dyad is indivisible – that we can no longer speak of the patient or the therapist as 'individuals', as though they are not always in relation to one another. It also questions the differences between the 'inner' world and the 'outer' world, as they may be more intertwined than we are used to thinking.

However, this is also true of the multi-personal relations of groups who meet for the purpose of psychotherapy. Group therapy is about close contact between participants in an emotional 'field' who will be unconsciously and consciously pulled and pushed in such a way that personal and interpersonal characteristics 'like an assumption, will be co-created, maintained and worked through inter-subjectively by the linking objects' (Billow, 2003: 40).

Affects are embedded in a history of relations; emotions are shaped by reciprocal, though often asymmetrical influences. Mirroring, resonance and exchange can be understood as aspects of the intersubjective dialogue, which governs the development of communication in the family and groups. First the mother but later others, including, of course, the father, become intersubjective partners establishing patterns of relatedness that move and touch each other mutually by permeating one another's conscious and unconscious psyches.

Mind may be itself an intersubjective result of this traffic (Foulkes, 1975). Viewing a whole relational space called the Mind, or a containing space, in which mutual thinking, exchanging and elaborating process is shared, may be one of the major contributions of the intersubjective 'turn'. While it may often be impossible to directly recognize the intersubjective influence of another's mind on one's own mind, and on the shared space by which a mind is defined, such unconscious interpersonal influence seems to be an essential element of the human condition. It may also be the basis of socio-cultural 'constraint' (Hopper, 1981).

Martin Weegmann has stressed that from an intersubjective perspective, both healthy and unhealthy psychological developments are in essence irreducibly relational. Contributions to the formation of this perspective have been made by many psychoanalysts, especially those who have emphasized the importance of projective and introjective processes in human relations, e.g. Ferenczi, Klein, Fairbairn, Winnicott and Balint, and more recently self-psychologists, such as Stolorow et al. (2002). It also seems important and natural to include Bion in this list of psychoanalysts who have contributed to the description of a relational frame of reference, especially with respect to his (Bion, 1963) model of container/contained.

Relational thinking may innovate perspectives on processes thought to be mainly intrapersonal. An example could be the concept of shame, which is often considered a very individual feeling. Shame could be the result of an unconscious meeting with others, a kind of alarm system warning when the potential rejection of a group is activated. The participants' shame, aroused in any interaction, being intersubjectively connected, may be an unconscious alarm ignited by a possible societal expulsion. One's own contribution to this rejection mechanism we define as 'shame'.

Socio-cultural systems are constructed on the basis of what modern psychodramatists and socio-dramatists call the 'co-conscious' and the 'co-unconscious' (Weinberg, 2007). Persons in co-conscious and co-unconscious relationships co-create a shared 'third space' (Ogden, 1994) in which and through which 'social facts' such as societies and cultures and social systems more generally are represented. Group analysts conceptualize such social systems in terms of what we call 'dynamic' and 'foundational' matrices, which Lavie would describe as intersubjective notions. They are based on the idea that social systems are both more than the sum of their parts and more than the sum of their participants. The socio-cultural communicative structures of social systems, ranging from families to organizations to nations, are derived from these co-constructed relational phenomena. It would be interesting to ask if the opposite is also true: that co-conscious and co-unconscious processes can only be understood in the context of their dynamic and foundational matrices.

Through tracing the notion of the relational person implicit in Foulkes's (1990) work to the influence of Norbert Elias, Joshua Lavie emphasizes that Foulkes and group analysis in general have contributed significantly to the passage from thinking about people as closed individuals to thinking about them as open relational persons. This intersubjective perspective has a powerful impact on therapy in general and especially on group analysis, where it creates a new therapeutic paradigm by asserting that the therapist is not the exclusive therapeutic factor. All persons-in-relation-in-a-group are mutually healing.

Although 'the concept of mental processes . . . [as] . . . multipersonal seems hard to accept(Foulkes, 1975: 253), it is this conceptualization of a 'transpersonal' emotional movement that turns group analysis into one of the sources of intersubjective thinking. Foulkes (1964) calls it 'an endo-psychic common union between two people'.

Intersubjective aspects of pathology are also connected to Foulkes's concept of location (Foulkes, 1948; Nitzgen, 2010), an entirely intersubjective notion. 'The location of pathology is not found in any individual alone, nor is it entirely interpersonal, but to be looked at in his relationships' (Foulkes, 1948: 1). Similarly to the relational location of Mind, then the 'sick mind' of an individual or a group may be considered a 'relational pathology' (Friedman, 2013).

What influence does intersubjectivity have on group-analytic practice? Does it lead to a renewed combination of psychogenic and sociogenic aspects in the group-analytic work (Lavie, 2011)? Will the conductors of therapeutic groups have to develop a 'particular sensitivity' and should they 'leave things unresolved, in mid-air, incomplete (Foulkes (1964: 287) as Weegmann (2011) suggests? The conductor's complex position within the context of intersubjective approaches to clinical work should be discussed and practised, in order to understand even more fully what it means to be a 'conductor-in-the-group' rather than a therapist who mainly maintains distance from his patients. The 'intersubjective turn' casting new light on the concepts of neutrality and abstinence will probably influence our profession through mutual learning and a further development in our thinking.

Note

1 This chapter appeared previously as Friedman, R (2014) Group Analysis Today – Developments in Intersubjectivity. *Group Analysis*, 47(3) 194–200.

References

Billow, R.M. (2003) Relational Variations of the 'Container-Contained'. *Contemporary Psychoanalysis*, 39: 27–50.

Bion, W.R. (1963) *Elements of Psycho-Analysis*. London: William Heinemann. Reprinted London: Karnac Books. Reprinted in Seven Servants, 1977.

Foulkes, E. (Ed.). (1990) *S.H. Foulkes Selected Papers*. London: Karnac.

Foulkes, S.H. (1948) *Introduction to Group-Analytic Psychotherapy*. London: Heinemann.

Foulkes, S.H. (1964) *Therapeutic Group Analysis*. London: Allen and Unwin.

Foulkes, S.H. (1975) Problems of the Large Group. In E. Foulkes (Ed.), (1990) *S.H. Foulkes Selected Papers* (pp. 249–269). London: Karnac.

Freud, S. (1912) Ratschläge für den Arzt bei der psychoanalytischen Behandlung. Zentralblatt für Psycho-analyse. II: 483–489; *GW*, VIII: 376–387; 'Recommendations to Physicians Practising Psycho-Analysis', *SE*, 12: 111–120.

Friedman, M. and Vietze, P. (1972) The Competent Infant. *Peabody Journal of Education*, 49(4): 314–322.

Friedman, R. (2012) Dreams and Dreamtelling: A Group Approach. In J.L. Kleinberg (Ed.), *The Wiley-Blackwell Handbook of Group Psychotherapy* (First Edition, pp. 479–499). West Sussex, UK: John Wiley and Sons, 2011.

Friedman, R. (2013) Individual or Group Therapy? Indications for Optimal Therapy. *Group Analysis*, 46: 164–170.

Grotstein, J.S. (2002) 'We Are Such Stuff as Dreams Are Made on' – Annotations on Dreams and Dreaming in Bion's Works. In C. Neri, M. Pines and R. Friedman (Eds.), *Dreams in Group Psychotherapy* (pp. 110–146). London: Jessica Kingsley Publishers.

Hopper, E. (1981) *Social Mobility: A Study of Social Control and Insatiability*. Oxford: Blackwell. Excerpts reprinted in Hopper, E. (2003) *The Social Unconscious: Selected Papers*. London: Jessica Kingsley.

Hopper, E. (2003) *The Social Unconscious: Selected Papers*. London: Jessica Kingsley.

Husserl, E. (1931) *Cartesian Meditations: An Introduction to Phenomenology*. Translated by D. Cairns. Dordrecht: Kluwer, 1960.

Lavie, J. (2011) The Lost Roots of the Theory of Group Analysis: 'Interrelational Individuals' or 'Persons'. In E. Hopper and H. Weinberg (Eds.), *The Social Unconscious in Persons, Groups, and Societies. Volume 1: Mainly Theory* (pp. 155–178). London: Karnac.

Lawrence, W.G. (2007) *Infinite Possibilities of Social Dreaming*. London: Karnac Books.

Mitchell, S.A. (1988) *Relational Concepts in Psychoanalysis*. Cambridge, MA and London: Harvard University Press.

Nitzgen, D. (2010) Hidden Legacies. S.H. Foulkes, Kurt Goldstein and Ernst Cassirer. *Group Analysis*, 43: 354–371.

Ogden, T. (1994) The Analytical Third: Working With Intersubjective Clinical Facts. *International Journal of Psychoanalysis*, 75(1): 3–20.

Rafaelsen, L. (1996) Projections, Where Do They Go? *Group Analysis*, 29: 143–158.

Redl, F. (1942) Group Emotion and Leadership. *Psychiatry*, 5: 573–596.

Stolorow, R.D., Atwood, G.E. and Orange, D.M. (2002) *Worlds of Experience: Interweaving Philosophical and Clinical Dimensions in Psychoanalysis.* New York: Basic Books.

Weegmann, M. (2011) Working Intersubjetively: What Does It Mean for Theory and Therapy? In E. Hopper and H. Weinberg (Eds.), *The Social Unconscious in Persons, Groups, and Societies. Volume 1: Mainly Theory* (pp. 133–154). London: Karnac.

Weinberg, H. (2007) So What Is This Social Unconscious Anyway? *Group Analysis*, 40(3): 307–322.

Winnicott, D.W. (1958) Anxiety Associated With Insecurity. In *Through Pediatrics to Psycho-Analysis* (pp. 97–100). London: Tavistock.

PART III

The soldier's matrix, or how to live with existential anxieties, trauma and hopes for glory. The encounter with conflict in communities through the sandwich model – a combination between small and large groups to heal society

INTRODUCTION TO PART III

Introduction

The soldier's matrix

I live in a society which is always felt to be in some kind of existential danger. Many would agree that the reality is felt as threatening, for example the months before the Six-Day War or the first two weeks of the Yom Kippur War. But this is also true for Israelis' emotional reactions to annihilation anxiety (Hopper, 2003) resulting from threats of Hezbollah's and Iran's leaders. In my society there are also moments of great elation and pride, identifications which feel so glorious that they seem to merit dying for. War victories, solidarity, selfless sacrifices and the feeling of not being alone are part of the glory of the matrix, which alongside anxiety and existential threats are very much part of our emotional, everyday life. These emotional processes cause massification processes in our society which also translate into a progressively diminishing guilt, shame and empathy. I consider all of these to be the main traits of the soldier's matrix (Friedman, 2015), where everyone is enrolled in a selfless, heroic and sacrificing manner. When I refer to the social unconscious of our Matrix here, I mean that perspectives or views of the individual matrix, our foundation culture and the present 'dynamic' matrix co-create a complex, unconscious field. This tri-partite model is at the heart of the soldier's matrix (Friedman, 2018) – the culture of a society under the stress of existential threat and hopes for glory. Individuals are enlisted as a soldier for decades (we serve 30 years of one month every year), which helps to give acceptance to the notion that soldiers are only society's delegates, while everyone, including women, children and the elderly, are enrolled and serving. While it seems that today it is easy to serve 'the cause' without any reflection, for those who are able to reflect, the Israeli Army and its warlike situations are an interesting space to investigate ambiguity. A connected subject is society's and the parent's proud willingness to sacrifice one's own children by sending them into combat.

But only after meeting Germans in Germany, encountering their positions in what I call the anti–soldier's matrix, could I have insights about myself as well as the social and emotional process around me. Unfortunately, the Israeli soldier's matrix is rapidly developing in the frightening direction of the German soldier's matrix. Neighbouring matrices also influence each other, and so, children of some of my Arab patients pray for a strong Israeli army that can defend them from Daesh (ISIS). My interpretation of this is that the Arab population in Israel are also part of the Israeli soldier's matrix.

Living in a soldier's matrix also means being exposed to influences which invade personal boundaries and what we call the 'transpersonal' way of communicating through the individual. The culture of the soldier's matrix seems to hold a monopoly on the individual's mind and to expect resilience and selflessness in the struggle for survival or the fight for glory. Invariably this culture will restrict personal development because of the pressure in the Large Group to identify with the rather rigid norms of society. Together with the reduction of violence-inhibitors like shame and guilt, more hate and scapegoating will be observed – together with a tendency to blindly follow a leadership which will seem fit to 'save' society from its enemies.

Much of my present understanding stems from participating and conducting large groups. The social matrix seems more visible and graspable when 40 or more people sit down in circles and try to monologue and dialogue. Especially if the groups are working through time, and can cope with a reduced 'inclusion security', which differentiates them from small groups and allows a clearer reflection of societal processes.

Is total defeat necessary for a nation to cope with its soldier's matrix, as with the German experience? How can one elaborate the enormous influences the soldier's matrix has on society and the individual? In my search for tools that enable some working-through of these emotional tendencies I designed the sandwich model (Friedman, 2016), a setting which combines small and large groups. Applying it in different communities, we found it efficiently coping with annihilation anxiety, glory and 'authority relations'. One of the most important processes in the sandwich model is the ability of individuals and subgroups to 'distance' themselves from their soldier's matrix and make it possible to reflect on the processes happening. Thus, it seems possible that the sandwich model is a setting which heals society from a monopolizing and limiting society. It helped me to grow personally, and to enter into a dialogue which achieves not only separation, but also affiliation.

References

Friedman, R. (2015) A Soldier's Matrix: A Group Analytic View of Societies in War. *Group Analysis*, 48(3): 239–257.

Friedman, R. (2016) The Group Sandwich Model for International Conflict Dialog. Using Large Groups as a Social Developmental Space. In S.S. Fehr (Ed.), *101 Interventions in Group Psychotherapy* (pp. 83–85). New York: Routledge.

Friedman, R. (2018) Beyond Rejection, Glory and the Soldier's Matrix: The Heart of My Group Analysis [42nd Foulkes Lecture]. *Group Analysis*, 51(4): 389–405.

Hopper, E. (2003) Incohesion: Aggregation/Massification; The Fourth Basic Assumption in the Unconscious Life of Groups and Group-like Social Systems. In R.M. Lipgar and M. Pines (Eds.), *Building on Bion: Roots*. London: International Library of Group Analysis 20, Jessica Kingsley Publishers.

7

A SOLDIER'S MATRIX

A group-analytic view of societies in war[1]

My soldier's matrix

In my early childhood I was confronted with violence. I often found myself between two frontlines, each of them affected by violence. On the one side I was surrounded by the 'attackers': the German frontliners who in spite of having to flee Germany, were still the German soldiers of the First World War, whom I perceived as somehow cold, irritated and ambivalent, near and far at the same time.

There was my Prussian grandfather, who used to show me his many war wounds. There was also my grand-uncle, also multiply wounded, who told me of his disappointment at how the Berlin Arians did not only not appreciate his performance as one of the first German tank commanders on the Russian frontline – but also expelled him from his work at the stock exchange and drove him out of Germany. I thought that they mourned their lost homeland and their lost culture more than their numerous lost family members whom they never mentioned.

On the other side were the victims of the Shoah – the survivors of my family – sharing their pain. With my aunts, uncles and cousins, recently arrived from the camps and a shattered Europe, I felt much more warmth. I felt loved, and I was told that they lived only for my cousins and me. However, I overheard their whispers, full of hatred and shame; they, too, were entangled in an inner war, and still felt responsible for the awful things they did or experienced in the camps. They were full of vengeance too, in particular towards Kapos. For me, the victims' and soldiers' injuries were incompatible. When, as a child, I tried to cope with war, playing cowboys and Indians or Hitler against Churchill, my grandfather was easily angered. Like many post-traumatized people, he could not stand playfulness, and accused me of enacting my aggression. Could it be that already back then, I was unconsciously positioning myself in the soldier's matrix? I started to ask myself: are soldiers sick?

During the preparation of this article it was inevitable for me to confront my own experiences in war. Thus I had endless thoughts on the question of the soldier's pathology: for example: while going from an ambush over to an attack, do all comrades react uniformly in having to run into a hail of bullets? Of course not: soldiers do not follow commands uniformly. Although you would hope for all of them to get up immediately and run with you, there is usually only a little group of a few soldiers running with you on the frontline. A so-called second row of comrades, getting up more slowly, will run behind you whilst you hope that they do not use their guns on you. There is also a third line, the group of soldiers who seem to have had a hard time getting up – they follow at a distance. I often asked myself: which of these are the healthier?

The matrix

According to S.H. Foulkes, the matrix is the hypothetical web of relationships on four levels of communication.

> The individual participates in its formation and creation and at the same time re-establishes the conditions of his own primary network as experienced. . . . The matrix is the common shared ground which ultimately determines the meaning and significance of all events.
>
> *(Foulkes, 1964: 292)*

Subgroups vary in their identification levels with the matrix, which influences their emotional relations to outside enemies. The matrix's high permeability renders it also extremely exposed to the inter- and transpersonal flow of communication and emotions, and also makes for a strong environment's influence. The latent and manifest flow of information between matrix members applies also to the family, which, like a group, may lead to the matrix's best but possibly also worst destructiveness.

By the term 'soldier' I mean more than just the delegated man in uniform. It includes the humans' mental and physical experiences at war, and the influence on all members of the matrix. Terror subgroups may be defined as a soldier's matrix; a female suicide bomber is like a soldier, but her whole human environment – women, children, the old – must probably also be that of a 'soldier' of a war matrix. All it needs is anxiety, hatred and most likely a 'truth' which may further condense feelings. A soldier's matrix does not need a state, as Norbert Elias (1989) thought it to be. The state seems to have lost its monopoly for violence a long time ago, and it can be seen more as a reciprocal influence between individuals and masses, as well as weapons and identities, all creating emotions which result in warring activities. Soldiers, freedom fighters or terrorists only execute the delegated violence of the matrix.

The relationship between the individual and its matrix can also be represented by Foulkes's category of personification, which means that individuals can stand in for subconscious processes, and voice or act them (out). Personification or delegation is a very complex phenomenon; identification and projective identification processes may be responsible for the many shades of the different soldier's matrices, being part of the same process of mutual influence (Rafaelsen, 1996). Of course, the bigger the existential threat and the closer the danger of a conflict, the stronger the influence of the matrix on all members and subgroups. We can also witness this process in school classes, Facebook and many social organizations where monolithic thinking and massification phenomena (Hopper, 2003) may in many cases dominate the group's Mind.

The implicit and often partly subconscious target of the group is its efficiency: in addition to needing others – a group or an organization – to perform wherever one cannot achieve an aim alone, it should be as able, competent and successful as possible. Being part of the best group increases the possibility to survive, to win a game or to play the most wonderful music. The efficiency function interplays with the individual's dependency on the group subordinating his personal motivations to social influences. Tom Ormay's concept of Nos for the so-called group instinct is a useful conceptualization of this side: 'One is none' (Ormay, 2013).

Given this natural tendency to belong to the best group implies that groups undertake significant efforts of selection, hoping to insure and develop their efficiency. Such a selection process may lead to the group's better functioning, but it may also result in destructive processes which may harm individuals or subgroups that are perceived as superfluous or even dangerous in the face of an existential threat to the matrix. Individuals or subgroups do marginalize, exclude or even eliminate others. There seems to be a qualitative distinction between marginalization, which means exclusion, and rejection, which depicts expulsion and destruction. In our collective unconscious, being rejected from a significant group emotionally still means death by expulsion to the desert or coldness.

The example of the sluggish soldiers delaying their charge also raises the question of the influence in the matrix. The continuum between the total dominance of the group on the individual to a possible individual 'free choice' has often been addressed. Here I talk about a semi-conscious process, which includes not only the relationship between soldiers and a dominating soldier's matrix, but also all other matrix members who take part in any identification and efficiency process of the large group (Volkan, 2013).[2] Is it possible at all for the average human being to make a personal choice, even under the threat of being marginalized in the matrix, let alone destroyed? Would it be a development, a return to a different balance between the horizontal and the vertical, which is better and more precisely defined in group therapy than in social dynamics and the large group?

The important theoretical discussion on the relationship between the (soldier's) matrix and the 'social unconscious' (Hopper and Weinberg, 2011) and the 'collective unconscious' (Mies, 2007; Scholz, 2014) cannot be dealt with in this article. I also will not discuss soldier's trauma or the traumas of societies in and after war. Instead, I would rather try to get an understanding of the 'normal' relationship between the soldier and his society, which may all be 'enlisted' in their matrix struggle.

The group-analytic emotional attitude to the group

S.H. Foulkes started his group-analytic patient groups out of clinical curiosity; he intuited a curative influence of relationships. Interestingly enough, he was surprised how simply his group method could be translated to the soldier's matrix in Northfield, and then also to other matrices. This seemed to have strengthened his 'trust in the group', and the result was a more open and less anxious Foulkesian attitude to the group.

While 'trust the group' is a complicated statement, this attitude is fundamentally different in group analysis than the subliminal fear of the group we can see with other approaches. The friendlier group-analytic approach of the conductors to the matrix helps to reduce the anxieties of the members in small and large groups. Foulkes (1975c) even went further to say that some of the extreme dramatic movements in large groups are 'conductor-made': 'It is in the hands of the conductor to make this more or less dramatic, not to say traumatic' (Foulkes, 1975c: 265).

For a long time, the difference between individual, small and large group therapy was not well understood. The Northfield experience has proven that, while the social web, i.e. the (soldier's) matrix, can be treated, the large group still terrifies individuals. Could this be the reason that small group therapy maintained a monopoly in the group-analytic practice?[3]

The complex relations to violence in the foundation matrix are intriguing. For example: 'Thou shalt not kill' does not seem to be applied in reality to the 'foundation matrix', which is the 'basic common ground (of communication and interaction and understanding) and is based on what was called *foundation matrix*' (Foulkes, 1975b: 291). Close and known humans should not be killed (like the prohibition to repeat Cain and Abel's murder); but political enemies and for the sake of one's own survival, i.e. in a situation where the soldier's matrix appears, a matrix influenced by war and schizoid-paranoid situations, you are obliged to kill the opponent group members. Murderous violence is not only legitimized, it also arouses collective unconscious strong defences against feelings of guilt, shame or empathy for the enemy's suffering. This is the essence of the film *The Act of Killing* (Oppenheimer, 2012), or, as Voltaire said, 'It is forbidden to kill; therefore murderers are punished, unless they kill in large numbers and to the sound of trumpets!'

The soldier's matrix in Israel

While writing this article it became increasingly clear to me that in Israel, we live in a soldier's matrix. Israel runs the risk of being attacked time and again. Men and women spend years as soldiers, the army's operations are well known and an open and unspoken knowledge of the war is everywhere. Information as well as the emotional aspects of living under threat are shared not only by uniformed units but by the whole population. Thus, at the time of writing this article, the local experience provides for many of the understandings gained here (July–August 2014). One of many examples would be the collective identification with stigmatizing the enemy: the absolute security that there is no possibility to negotiate with those who attacked one's own cities before; the denial of shame and guilt about the army's wrongdoing, and the diminishing of non–'politically correct' empathy.

Aggression in the large group and regression

Serge Moscovici writes in his book *The Age of the Crowd: A Historical Treatise on Mass Psychology* (1985) that mass communication influences the regression of the individual. Freud thought that, by feeling part of a mass, we regress as individuals. The mass turns us into neurotics. Moscovici believed that modern communication instantaneously produces a mass on the base of a common fantasy of the identification with a great number of individuals, which are in relation to each other.[4] Volkan (2013) writes about his concept of the 'large group Identity' in a similar way.

Kernberg (2003) points out that regression shows several characteristics: for example, the difficulty to think or a tendency of the mass to hate and envy the individual and individuality. Like Bion, he thinks that the large group can choose only one of two regressive paths: (1) the 'dependent basic assumption group', which he describes as a narcissistic-regressive group and (2) the 'flight-fight basic assumption group', where he observes a paranoid regression (Bion, 1962; Kernberg, 2003).

My question is: Can we really talk about regression in respect of the encounter of the individual with the large group, where actually the chronologic and the situational/characteristic conditions of regression do not exist? Do we have definitions of subgroup regressions? Does the whole large group or its relations regress? Could it be that the encounter with large groups and the influence of the mass cause totally different modes of interaction, which become manifest? Is it possible that the relationship with a large group results in a qualitative difference, which is not more or less regressive or progressive, but like water, which behaves completely differently as one drop than as part of a cloud or fog, just 10 minutes before? How fast can 'a very rapid regression of the ego to these early stages, to its very genesis' (Foulkes, 1975cc: 267) happen? I think change, which many have called regression, is not a regression, as it happens in seconds, it is not a 'dissociation' and should be defined as a different state of mind. The different understanding has a bearing on its possible transformation.

If we deal with regression, we have to treat it therapeutically – an approach I would challenge. Could we heal, for example, an Adolf Eichmann, who could neither be diagnosed as regressive or unthinking or only 'narcissistic' or 'totally dependent'? If we rather understand it as a different state of mind, we might use a more practice-based approach, like 'ego training in action' (Foulkes, 1968: 181).

Kernberg (2003) explains social violence with a pathologic leadership showing signs of malign narcissism or paranoia. Unstructured groups and masses exposed to massive propaganda will regress, split into subgroups, and by merging again into a large group, are able to bear physical extermination of de-humanized subgroups. By blaming only the leadership, we may be using defence mechanisms as a denial of the collective responsibility for violence.

The quick transformations in the large group's matrix violence are not necessarily regressive; they often seem to be evidence of unconscious fears and identification with authorities, a 'healthy' primary tendency to survive and a natural understanding of the large group matrix, and the need to collectively adapt to conflictual situations. Although it seems that these are not clear-cut processes, it seems important to better understand and investigate the underlying process. The term 'change of identity', conceptualized by the sociologist Reicher (1987), corresponds more with my understanding of large group dynamics than 'regression'. Most probably, the emotional pressure of the mass on the individual, which in group-analytic settings can be seen particularly in the early phases of the large group, immediately push the individual to give up parts of his or her personal identity in favour of fundamental identifications and counter-identifications with the large group. Even small children seem to be aware of how to behave in such a large group.

Another significant underlying mechanism of this dynamic is the 'two step' development of belonging: Humans long for inclusion (Schlapobersky, 2015), and in a first step they find it existentially important to belong to a group. In a second step they seem unconsciously anxious about being expelled from it and cling or submit to the matrix aims. In a split moment those fundamental human positions, states of mind are turned on like a mode rather than experiencing a 'regression' in the large group.

According to Moscovici, the medieval drummer transformed the villagers immediately into a large group by announcing the latest news. Though the modes of transferring information change, the impact of simultaneous information to a mass is tremendous. Radio, newspapers, television, Facebook and Twitter transform the large group culture in seconds.

In a soldier's matrix, the psychoanalytic approach would say that people's 'regressed self' is sometimes the target of psychoanalytic treatment, intervening at a level of personal childhood internalizations. It is common to see these remain intact in a private setting but completely change as a reaction to the large group situation and the mass. 'Ego-training in action' (Foulkes, 1964: 82) was already mentioned as another approach, and can also be applied to group-analytic large groups to practise movement on the continuum between Self and Nos. The participation in the large group setting facilitates subgroups' and individuals' reflection and habituation in their relations to the mass, the community and even the nation. Group analysis has in its hands a unique instrument, where the reciprocal influence in the matrix, including the conductors, can be 'played' with. It is our clinical experience that habituated participants in the large group are not only more aware of the social aspects of identity, but have a greater choice of dialogue with others and the mass.

Matrix and pathology of aggression in relations

Foulkes thought that the 'location' of all psychological diseases is not found inside individuals but in the space between related people (1948). Foulkes's opinion, that pathology is an interpersonal issue, makes sense to many clinicians, even if we are scared by the shared responsibility for the disorders of others. Two such interpersonal pathologies, which I call relation disorders, directly related to interpersonal violence, will be discussed. The first one happens when a matrix disinhibits aggression; the second is a disorder of relations marked by extreme violence both towards others and oneself, in the form of self-sacrifice, when behaving aggressively towards enemies. The rejection relation disorder shares many of the soldier's matrix characteristics, especially the reduced feelings of guilt, shame and empathy. While these emotions inhibit violence, their lack promotes the occurrence of murderous impulses, sadism and other forms of violence. In the second disorder, where the Self is disturbed, the matrix promotes the renunciation of one's own Self up to the justification of its sacrifice – usually in a sea of violence. The soldier's matrix is characterized by both these group phenomena: reduced violence-inhibiting mechanisms and the promotion of selfless relations. Fundamental and partly unconscious pathogenic emotions, e.g. feeling the danger of being rejected as well as the subsequent existential threats, have an elementary impact on our behaviour. The price for the use of defences against annihilation anxieties is often a loss of one's individuality, together with the loss of other social emotions like compassion, becoming 'over-identified' with a social cause and 'identification with the aggressor' (Freud, 1936), which are also easily detected in the soldier's matrix.

Only if the whole matrix as the 'location' of interpersonal aggression undergoes change will individuals and subgroups have a greater choice for the use of force and greater possibility to take responsibility against violence. Under such conditions, soldiers, their relatives and even the whole societal culture may slowly feel that they may be able to move away from the soldier's matrix towards more free relations. This may involve a distancing process, which is crucial in order to regain the lost capacity for guilt and shame about committed crimes, and the return of empathy for the victims. An example of this is Germany's post-war generation's enduring difficulty to contain painful late mourning and impotence processes from their recent history.

Relation disorders

Following Agazarian's research on the dynamics of group development (1994), with particular reference to four 'containing-roles', which carry mismanaged emotions in every stage, I made an attempt to describe four relation disorders. Rather than concentrating on the 'container's' pathology I considered the creation of a whole 'figuration' (Foulkes, 1948), a set of (disordered) relations involved in a group dynamic. We may also view these relation disorders as condenser phenomena, found almost exclusively in group interactions. They seem to require group therapy as their optimal treatment (Friedman, 2013). From the four I will concentrate here on two relevant relation disorders: the rejection disorder and the disorders of the self.

Rejection disorder

The 'Scapegoating Position' can be understood as a special group 'figuration', of interpersonal relations in groups that fail to contain violence. The relations between the scapegoats, who are afraid of being rejected. try everything to be able to belong to the group, and the 'scapegoaters', who develop partly unconscious dynamics of violence towards a (hated) group member or subgroup can become uncontained. As a result, the scapegoat may be rejected and eliminated. The dynamics of this pathological relation cannot occur without the existential need of the scapegoat for inclusion in the group, and his increasing willingness to accept violence against himself in order to avoid rejection. In this cyclic process, the scapegoater's motivation of selecting group members for rejection and expulsion – colludes with the scapegoat's unconscious need for belonging and an ever-growing fear of annihilation.

Dicks (1972) investigated German KZ-guards who were prisoners in England. Their main characteristics were twofold: their submission to the SS-authority with whom they identified on the one hand. They could execute their control over the prisoners in the camps, who were totally exposed to annihilation– cruelly and without any doubt or guilt. On the other hand this guiltless, shameless and 'empathy-less' psychopathic attitude of the scapegoaters happened only in a certain matrix. Dicks could prove that these people, who in their 'social system', which we could consider as the 'scapegoater-matrix' (or Rejection Disorder, Friedman, 2013), showed many signs of a severe personality disorder, were neither dangerous nor violent men elsewhere.[5] Perhaps you do not need pathology in order to become a psychopath, because the disorder depends on the matrix and the relations in the group. This may partly answer the question: How do soldiers get sick?

As a matter of fact, we all witness and even follow more hatred and violence in rejection matrices than we would like to admit. Harm Stehr (2013) described in a conference in Bonn an example of a typical classroom configuration, which could be called 'scapegoating position'. As a boy, he witnessed the rejection of a classmate. The group expelled a seemingly inferior and 'inappropriate' member, probably as the result of an efficiency process (as described earlier), which determines the selection process in the group. Again, groups tend to become elite troops, and as in sport, there are main players, bench players and those who were rejected from the team. In Stehr's recount, at that time, not one classmate identified with the victim and intervened. In fact, all of us feel relief not to become the scapegoat ourselves. In group-analytic therapy, we try to treat Disorders by working with all sides who are reciprocally involved in the relation disorder. We must address the interaction between unspoken rejection anxieties with the linked hatred and violence.[6]

The 'Scapegoating Position' goes beyond classic meanings of what was described in the decades after the Second World War as scapegoats, who are supposedly subjects of projections and even envy (Garland et al., 1973). Scapegoating includes not only hatred and destruction fantasies towards the weak and strong, but also rejection, extermination and death for the enemy, and a tendency to act the emotions out violently.[7] It also includes an unconscious relation with the scapegoat, who is unable to separate from the wish to belong to the perpetrator's group. The scapegoating position can produce a veritable 'hatred-training in action' (Foulkes,

1975bb, 'ego-training in action'). Examples of destructive processes in large groups are numerous: the German matrix before and after the Nuremberg discrimination laws and the expulsion of Hagar and Ismail to the desert are just a couple of them. The threat of rejecting all those Israeli 'traitors' who were critical in the last Gaza war, or even those who were not identified enough is another example of the 'scapegoating position'.

Relation disorders of the self

The second relation disorder discussed here describes pathological developments of the Self. When members over-identify with the matrix, men and women will subordinate their own interests and motivations to a need or will of the group. The symptoms of this loss of the self are gendered very differently: while women selflessly serve others, men sacrifice themselves, their lives, as 'heroes' (Agazarian, 1994) in conflicts. Selfless protagonists, men and women, are being educated or seduced to sacrifice the Self and enjoy significant support by 'selfish' fans.

Many of our patients, feeling depressed or living in omnipotent fantasies, suffer from this very relation disorder. Self-abandonment engenders violence by abuse of many subgroups of the matrix. Even survival in the group within such a matrix is conceived to be a selfless, suicidal soldier's devotion, which may be generalized to all men. In unconscious fantasies about father figures, the selfless soldier's devotion in order to defend their child and its perception, contributes to the child's development. A healthy 'primary paternal preoccupation', the equivalent to the 'primary maternal preoccupation' (Winnicott, 1956; Doron, 2014) can have significant supportive functions for the individual and his feeling of confidence in this world. Thus, social situations of Selflessness may have complex functions, which partly can be considered as 'normal'.

A dream may contain an example of 'typical' aggressive and suicidal tendencies in the selfless relation disorder:

During a conference organized by the IIGA (Israel Institute of Group Analysis) in the Kibbutz Eyn Gedi I pleaded, as a member of the large group, for a stronger feeling of security for our (Israeli) existence. I pointed out that only a feeling of security enables dialogue with the enemy. I said a sentence that hit me: 'We should stop living as if we are still at the gates of Auschwitz'. There were many reactions, but I myself felt great sadness: I had tackled a painful taboo.

The same night I had a vivid dream: The Arabs conquered Israel, we had lost the war and the enemy was all around us. I fled with my family into a wadi, a gorge. My children were small again, the same age as my grandchildren today. Everything was green, like the reality of the current winter. Other families were hiding with us. The situation became more dangerous, because the Syrian army was approaching, and I knew that there would be a 'bad end'. In order to protect my family, I decided to blow myself up on military installations, which looked like gas tanks, believing that this would stop the occupation. A Druze officer was willing to assist me. I remember the sad look in the eyes of my wife when I left. Luckily a twist of fate brought a rescuing army (I think they were Russians, like at the gates of Auschwitz).

It goes without saying that such a dream has many possible meanings. I would like to emphasize here the tendency to self-sacrifice, which for men does not seem pathological, but rather natural. Questions of sacrifice, which can be included under the self relation disorders, are all over this article. From my grandfather's and uncle's heroic sacrifices in the First World War to women who find it crucially important to mother the next generation of soldiers, sacrifice in dreams and reality is a central aspect of the soldier's matrix. Are soldiers sick? Kamikaze pilots wearing hats in their suicidal flight and other ambivalences toward Selflessness, make it clear that while renouncing on one's Self easily immerses soldiers and the whole population into an ocean of violence, it may still be a natural aspect of the family's and the community's life.

The Relation between Germany and the Soldier's Matrix – or: What Happened to Early Identifications? Let me share with you, very carefully, some thoughts about the German matrix today and the post-war years of the soldier's matrix. Sometimes an outsider, who is nevertheless related to a matrix, may bring some different elements into the discussion.

In Israel, the 'Nakbah', the Palestinian tragedy of the refugees, is an example of being part of our soldier's matrix, and influences it. This influence contains an often pre-conscious wish to prohibit its existence. While it is very easy to accept oneself as a victim, one of the most difficult psychological processes is to accept the fact that we all are also perpetrators. We may live in Haifa or Tel-Aviv, but we unconsciously share something with refugees in camps in Amman and Beirut, to which we are connected. No one in this land is really exempted, because the matrix contains everything: the evil, the less evil and the good. But being in a soldier's matrix actually means that these influences are fought and split off. The results of these splitting processes are panic or avoiding responses to any attempt of mature coping with the refugee problem. Similarly, most analysts of the last elections in Israel agree that they were won by the Likud through arising the annihilation fears awakened by the 'threatening masses of Arab voters driven in by the left'.[8] Annihilation anxiety is a driving motor in any soldier's matrix.

Until quite recently, the German matrix could be considered as a soldier's matrix. If we believe in unconscious interpersonal communication, it is clear that the entire soldier's matrix knew about the perpetrators as well as the victims, both about those involved in the making of the Shoah, as well those suffering from the bombardment of German cities. Frontline and home may be distant geographically, but as could be observed in the German debate about the 'Wehrmacht – Exposition' from the year 2001, there was no clear separation line in the war between civilians and the army, including army units like the SS – they were all part of the same matrix. But even after the war, the lack of distance and enmeshment in the soldier's matrix was omnipresent – even the identification with the Nazi system lasted for at least another 20 years. The soldier's matrix survived the 'purification' and other efforts to separate from the caused horror. Having said this, I certainly do not think the soldier's matrix alone can explain all the atrocities of the Holocaust. Many other societies in war and stress lived in soldiers' matrices that did not produce this extreme destructiveness.

The anti–soldier matrix?

The taboo of uniformed men, which seems to exist in Germany, questions the results of the processing of violence in the present matrix. A whole generation, after the 1960s, seems to have gone through a strong emotional movement from the soldier's matrix to an anti–soldier's matrix – probably a necessary process to cause a rupture with former identifications. Similarly to other societies, de-identification opens the gates to a different matrix, where shame and guilt feelings, fundamentally inter-generationally *inherited*, are allowed and elaborated. It is the next generation who suffers for the generations before them: 'The fathers eat sour grapes, and the children's teeth are set on edge' (Ezekiel 18.2.). The moving away from former identifications *may* be achieved through a de-idealizing of the relationship to German soldiers, which functions as a damaged container of prohibited libidinous desires. Transforming every former identification, once felt in the soldier's matrix, into objects of de-identification probably has educational and socializing functions. This hypothesis about the change in identifications may be further understood through group-analytic groups.

The soldiers who fought in a matrix that legitimized violence up to 1945 were not able to handle their own destructivity in the post-war period. Holdger Plata said, 'The life of many children of war was contaminated twice. It was determined by the experiences of the war- and post-war-time as well as from the first two decades of the German Federal Republic' (2004: 220). I interpret this statement as: the first 20 years after the Second World War were still determined by the matrix of the returned soldiers and the German war Habitus (Elias, 1989). The society continued to deny shame and guilt. It was only during the 1960s that a development of empathy could begin. Only then could the next generation start, consciously and unconsciously, to feel guilty for crimes done and stop hiding from the world because of a 'collective shame'. Only then could people start to distance themselves from the 'nation', from their parents, their neighbourhoods, the army and the education system – changing their own matrix. Summarising many conversations that I have had over the last few years with Germans, (individually and in group sessions) about this distancing process from the soldier's matrix, I would say:

The denial of army and war seems more often a schizoid paranoid (and not a depressive) attempt to escape the former soldier's matrix. It also includes thoughts of patricide, the taking revenge on the parents and sometimes the rage of defilement. But also, the contrary can be observed with many German children of perpetrators: the (often unconscious) identification with the parent's anxiety of being accused of war crimes leads to a suppression of the whole history by the taboo of the soldier's matrix. Generally splits and distancing from parents as an effort of 'purification' (Volkan, 2013) is a basic defence against shame and guilt. Finally, de-identification can also be a more or less unconscious attempt to stop the soldier's matrix of aggression pathology of countless previous generations. Dreams told in group analysis often teach us about these complex processes. Dreaming and dreamtelling open opportunities to try, simultaneously, two approaches to the exciting and the threatening: distancing from evil by purification processes, together with an effort to bridge splits and open up to difficult feelings.

Processes of de-identification are one of the most important promoters of societal development. De-identification has a similar significant function of separation as in the mother-child dyad. The more cohesive the matrix, the more complicated is the separation from the soldier's matrix. The betrayal of the former (post-traumatic) generation and a possible loss of 'primal paternal concern' are discussed. Fathers (and often mothers), who were part of soldiers' groups, who shared the terror of war experiences, expected solidarity from the next generation.

Thus we can understand what an enormous psychic achievement the generation born after the war accomplished by the de-identification of the German soldier's matrix. Shame, guilt and empathy could only be re-introduced by the younger generation.

In Germany, de-identification led to the fact that 'non-provocative' civil employees kept watch on military barracks. This transformed uniformed soldiers in a 'provocation', and thus a real threat to the new German identity. These issues may be optimally reflected upon in groups, where these often violent emotions originate, and where denied feelings may be worked through.

Transformation

Soldiers are neither sicker nor healthier than the matrix they live in. The power delegated to them by the matrix exists by a kind of consensus, especially when fighting external enemies. The split between a civil society and a soldier's matrix does not exist, and the stronger the democracy in war-stricken zones, the greater are the possibilities of a dialogue between the civil and militarized components of the soldier's matrix. Continuing splits, like in Northern Ireland for example, need conflict dialogue, in which 'enemies' meet for the purpose of getting to know the other side and speak with it. Acknowledging hardships in the presence of both sides renews a place for empathy. Political agreements and laws will not stop the soldier's matrix from dominating the culture of people nor prevent its return.

In 2013 I worked with Northern Irish rivalling parties, who called the situation 'unfinished business'. They had invited the IDI[9] to organize a meeting between political and civil society representatives of all colours, as well as police and paramilitaries. The title emphasizes that the soldier's matrix does not cede just because there is political agreement. It may take generations to stop social conflicts, and it may not really ever stop without interventions in which dialogue is introduced and structured. Direct encounters make this more possible, while distance reinforces splits and de-humanization. In different areas of conflict I have learned that a combination between personal encounters, integrated in small and large group work, may cause dramatic transformations. Personal encounters alone are rarely enough, and have to be supported by conflict dialogue in small groups, complemented by (not too) large groups to facilitate communication between social identities. Because in the end it is the matrix which dominates the individual's emotional modes of thought, the dialogue process has to be supported by participating in large groups that are more able to change the matrix culture through separating it from the soldier's matrix.

The group-analytic large group provides the space where we can learn to deal with identifications and the social fundamental fear of being rejected by society. Thus the large group provides us with the possibility to learn and to practise separation from authority. Maybe the best remedy for a democratic education is the mentioned 'ego-training-in action' in large groups; it could cause a move on the continuum between merging with the large group identity and total separation, isolation and rejection anxieties. In every soldier's matrix there is always a strong demand for identification. Practising in group-analytic large groups though could strengthen the courage to self-expression, which would sometimes make de-identification possible. In the short term it leads to paranoid confrontations between group members and authorities. In the long term it may allow the freedom to provocation and rebellion, which may also inhibit institutional violence. Transformation can also be achieved by civil and political leaders, who potentially serve as models for collective tolerance of institutionalized violence. A handshake, like Rabin's with Arafat, can change a lot. Unfortunately, politicians can also be models for hatred, revenge and distancing. For that reason it may be wiser to encourage long-term investment in complex group-analytic group work.

Notes

1 This chapter appeared previously as Friedman, R. (2015). A Soldier's Matrix: A Group Analytic View of Societies in War. *Group Analysis*, 48(3) 239–257.

2 Volkan's 'large group' implies often a nation, or entities on the base of identification. In this article I will differentiate it from the large group, which is a setting of many dozens up to hundreds of participants who meet for a session with one or more conductors (Wilke, 2014; Friedman, 2012).

3 Was this the reason why Elias was forgotten for so long and de Maré (de Maré, Piper and Thompson, 1991) marginalized? For example, the group-analytic attitude towards mental illness is still dominated by the individual, and marginalizes social and relation disorders.

4 Hopper (2003) thinks the mass influences into two directions: massification and aggregation, merging and fragmenting.

5 All of them did not suffer from any family trauma, but were people who grew up with a then 'normal' education, like most of us.

6 A personal note: as a child, I could unconsciously identify with my mother's scapegoat side. A few years ago we went back with her to Zerbst (a small town about 60 km south of Berlin) where she grew up, where this trait became understandable. She was born in 1923. At the age of 12 she was expelled from school, experiencing this probably as a rejection like in Harm Stehr's class. Later she was also banned from the houses of her two last German girlfriends with whom she would meet after school, and in which their socialist fathers had returned broken from concentration camps. 'Rita'chen, you cannot come anymore' they would say – probably out of fear from the scapegoaters, not because of hatred. After 1936 the social situation got even worse with the decrees of 'Aryan sports'. My mother

told us how she was banned from every sport; at the very end she was only allowed to play Ping-Pong, until this Asian sport became Aryan. Social rejection is a scar in the scapegoat for life, and in the rejecter, e.g. in soldiers, it can produce lifelong hatred.

7 See: The Act of Killing

8 www.slate.com/blogs/the_slatest/2015/03/17/netanyahu_arab_voters_at_polls_in_droves.html

9 IDI, International Dialogue Initiative, see www.internationaldialogueinitiative.com

References

The Act of Killing. (2012) Director: Joshua Oppenheimer. Distributed by Final Cut for Real, Worldwide. Voltaire. www.quotationspage.com/quote/30833.html

Agazarian, Y.M. (1994) The Phases of Group Development and the Systems-Centered Group. In V.L. Shermer and M. Pines (Eds.), *Ring of Fire* (pp. 36–86). London: Routledge.

Bion, W.R. (1962) *Learning From Experience*. London: William Heinemann. Reprinted Seven Servants, 1977.

de Maré, P., Piper, R. and Thompson, S. (1991) *Koinonia: From Hate, Through Dialogue to Culture in the Large Group*. London: Karnac Books.

Dicks, H.V. (1972) *Licensed Mass Murder: A Socio-Psychological Study of Some SS Killers*. London: Heinemann.

Doron, Y. (2014) Primary Maternal Preoccupation in the Group Analytic Group. *Group Analysis*, 47(1): 17–29.

Elias, N. (1989) *The Germans: Power Struggles and the Development of Habitus in the Nineteenth and Twentieth Centuries*. New York: Columbia University Press.

Foulkes, S.H. (1948) *Introduction to Group Analytic Psychotherapy*. London: Heinemann. Maresfield Reprint, Karnac Books: London, 1991.

Foulkes, S.H. (1964) *Therapeutic Group Analysis*. London: Karnac.

Foulkes, S.H. (1968) Group Dynamic Processes and Group Analysis. In E. Foulkes (Ed.), *Selected Papers of S.H. Foulkes: Psychoanalysis and Group Analysis* (pp. 175–185). London: Karnac, 1990.

Foulkes, S.H. (1975a) The Leader in the Group. In E. Foulkes (Ed.), *Selected Papers of S.H. Foulkes: Psychoanalysis and Group Analysis*. London: Karnac, 1990.

Foulkes, S.H. (1975b) *Group Analytic Psychotherapy: Method and Principles*. Gordon and Breach, Reprinted London: Karnac, 1986, 1991.

Foulkes, S.H. (1975c) Problems of the Large Group. In E. Foulkes (Ed.), *Selected Papers* (pp. 259–269). Karnac: London, 1990.

Freud, A. (1936) *The Ego and the Mechanisms of Defense* (Vol. 2). London: Karnac, 1992.

Friedman, R. (2012) Conducting a Large Group: Is It 'Informative' or Is It Also 'Transformative'? Comments to Teresa von Sommaruga Howard's Large Group in New Zealand. *Group Analysis*, 45(2): 263–268.

Friedman, R. (2013) Individual or Group Therapy? Indications for Optimal Therapy. *Group Analysis*, 46(2): 164–170.

Garland, J., Jones, H. and Kolodny, R. (1973) A Model for Stages of Development in Social Work Groups. In S. Bernstein (Ed.), *Exploration in Group Work* (pp. 17–71). Boston: Milford House.

Hopper, E. (2003) *Traumatic Experience in the Unconscious Life of Groups*. London: Jessica Kingsley Publishers.

Hopper, E. and Weinberg, H. (2011) *The Social Unconscious in Persons, Groups and Societies: Volume 1: Mainly Theory*. London: Karnac.

Kernberg, O. (2003) Sanctioned Social Violence: A Psychoanalytic View, Part I. *International Journal of Psychoanalysis*, 2003(84): 683–698.

Mies, T. (2007) Der Unterschied in der Gruppe. Heterogenität in der Gruppenpsychotherapie. *Gruppenpsychotherapie und Gruppendynamik*, 43: 21–33.

Ormay, T. (2013) *The Social Nature of Persons: One Person Is No Person*. London: Karnac.

Platta, H. (2004) Zwischen zwei Fronten – immer noch? Anmerkungen zur 'Kriegskinder' – Debatte und zur Rolle der 68er Generation in ihr. S. 211–126. In H. Radebold (Ed.), *Kindheiten im Zweiten Weltkrieg und ihre Folgen*. Giessen: Psychosozial-Verlag.

Rafaelsen, L. (1996) Projections, Where Do They Go? *Group Analysis*, 29(2): 143–158.

Reicher, S.D. (1987) Crowd Behaviour as Social Action. In J.C. Turner, M.A. Hogg, P.J. Oakes, S.D. Reicher and M.S. Wetherell (Eds.), *Rediscovering the Social Group: A Self-Categorization Theory* (pp. 171–202). Oxford: Basil Blackwell.

Schlapobersky, J.R. (2015) *From the Couch to the Circle: The Routledge Handbook of Group-Analytic Psychotherapy*. London: Routledge.

Scholz, R. (2014) (Foundation-) Matrix Reloaded – Some Remarks on a Useful Concept and Its Pitfalls. *Group Analysis*, 47(3): 201–212.

Stehr, H. (2012) Lecture at the D3G Conference. Bonn.

Stehr, H. (2013) Wege und Auswege von Hass und Destruktivität in Gruppen. *Gruppenpsychotherapie und Gruppendynamik*, 49(4): 331–349.

Volkan, V.D. (2013) *Enemies on the Couch: A Psychopolitical Journey Through War and Peace* (pp. 138–139). Durham, NC: Pitchstone Publishing.

Wilke, G. (2014) The Large Analytic Group and Its Conductor. In G. Wilke (Ed.), *The Art of Group Analysis in Organisations: The Use of Intuitive and Experiential Knowledge* (pp. 83–128). London: Karnac.

Winnicott, D.W. (1956) Primary Maternal Preoccupation. In D.W. Winnicott (Ed.), *Through Pediatrics to Psycho-Analysis*. London: Tavistock Publications, 1958.

8

THE GROUP SANDWICH MODEL[1] FOR INTERNATIONAL CONFLICT USING LARGE GROUPS AS A SOCIAL DEVELOPMENTAL SPACE[2]

Introduction

The sandwich model is designed to cope with conflictual situations in disturbed communities. It combines the relative security of small groups with the social character of large groups. Using the opportunities large groups can offer as the setting which offers the maximum face-to-face encounter possible, 80–300 and even more right-conducted participants can establish a unique social dialogue. Such powerful verbal and especially non-verbal experience exposes the participants to the views of others, as well as enables the ability to voice one's own view. The large group interaction, sandwiched between two small group sessions may have a unique potential to transform hate into co-existence and stop violence. The magic of seeing and feeling each other together with the development of a dialogue seems especially important after the failure of social media to cope with conflict.

Humans, being predominantly social, are deeply motivated by inclusion, exclusion and rejection dynamics. The different interpersonal settings, from dyads to small and large groups, are potential spaces which provide for differential coping necessities in relations. Moving to small groups, which unconsciously still hold the familiar promise of defending against exclusion or rejection, may give participants the possibility to feel secure while starting to voice conflicts. Then the LG, large group, with its completely different atmosphere may well provide for an unique opportunity to voice conflict and have a dialogue in the less secure social group. If it is possible to facilitate the LG to air questions of positions inside the group, or rejection and possible expulsion from the group and extermination, together with other, more specific anxieties and hate – it will be a start for the working through of the conflict. Moving back from the LG to a short small group, the sandwich model provides for a further opportunity to understand and cope with social dynamics of splitting and hating.

Selfless attitudes, together with societal and authoritarian dominance can be elaborated. The LG, this uncanny space, surrounded by the relative personal intimate security of the SG, small groups, may be the optimal place to dialogue with extremism and fanaticism. We need a FaceLOOK, in which violence-inhibiting mechanisms like guilt, shame and empathy can operate, contrary to the FaceBOOK, where virtual emotional distance makes endless fights possible. Finding a voice and the right tone in the presence of the threatening 'mass' and learning in the LG to move from a boundary-less chaos to a dialogue with mass and authority are developmental achievements.

The population

The model has been applied to both professionals and laypersons in conflicts, e.g. in the Ukraine during the war, in Northern Ireland, with politicians and leaders of the civil society and in German-Jewish dialogues. In schools, in whole villages and kibbutzim, where non-professional participants learned the SG Model and especially the LG 'tweeting' language. Participants' minimum age may be lower than we think – right now as my experience is with no less than individuals of 15 years old.

The intervention

When the dozen of conductors arrived in the village, about a hundred participants were waiting for us. For a while they were on the verge of violence following a dispute over accepting former enemies to live amongst them.

In the introduction (15 min.) the sandwich model and its advantages and difficulties was explained to participants and encouraged to commit to a 'working alliance' to the programme. The SG as a preparation for the LG was explained, together with the aims of the LG and possible anxieties: to communicate freely worries and aims in short tweets which aim to a dialogue.

Small groups (1 hour) helped the participants to find their voice and a kind of preliminary openness to diverging opinions.

After that a large group (1 hour and 10 minutes) of all 11 groups, together with their conductors, was formed. In this LG many of the community's socio-political positions were voiced in a very personal, emotional tone. This experience aroused both very strong feelings together with the awareness of differing and similar views and the danger of acting-out angry and opposing feelings.

After a pause (20 min.) a very short small group session (30 min.) had the function of calming down those who felt threatened by the LG. It also provided for an additional space in which to voice yet unspoken issues. A closure session of 15 minutes, in which attempts of voicing more significant contributions seemed possible, which thus finished the intervention.

Groups were led by highly professional conductors toward thinking and digesting some of the main problems in the village. They were encouraged to 'tweet' instead of monologuing. All conductors shared the group-analytic approach that large groups are not necessarily potentially psychotic and may be facilitated to constructive and honest dialogue. In some interventions the SG are led by trained members of the organization, who learn to provide a secure space for airing conflicts in the community.

General client responses

The vast majority of the participants of such sandwich model intervention wrote surprisingly favourable feedback. While many felt at first overwhelmed by the massive 'groupishness' of the evening and especially by the LG, unknown to the general

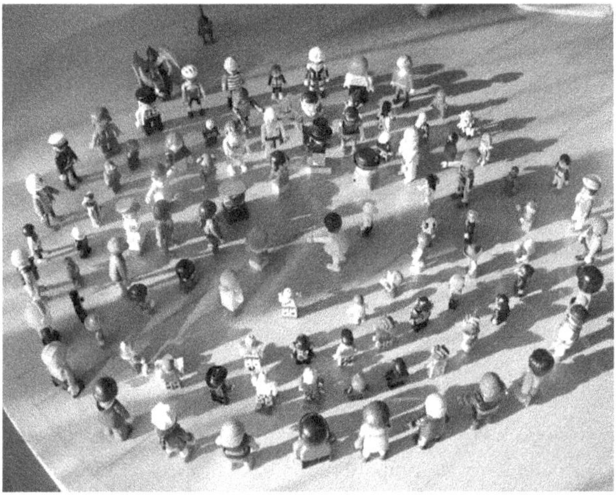

FIGURE 8.1 Large group meeting in concentric circles

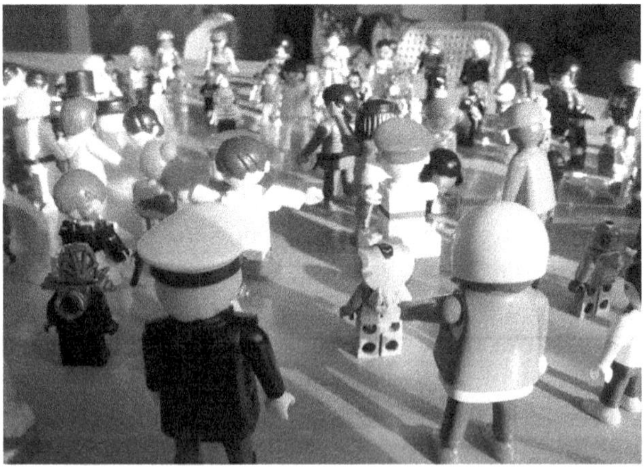

FIGURE 8.2 The setting which offers the maximum face-to-face encounter possible

population, many wrote about their awareness of the community's conflict and rifts. The developmental process ignited by the sandwich model continued in the following days and weeks. I think it takes sometimes months to understand the power of the sandwich model intervention. The most important feedback was that violence did not return for at least a year.

Conclusion

Legal accords (like high court rulings or 'the good Friday agreement') still leave communities who have to live with 'others' vulnerable to their traditional enmities, difficult stereotypes and tendencies to split and reject. In order to cope with the 'unfinished business' the sandwich model may be a very good solution if adopted as an ongoing process to be applied in the community.

Contraindications

The large group is a complicated interaction for the participants and has to be led accordingly by professional conductors who have a constructive approach to the LG. Although the individual's acquaintance with masses seems natural, for many participants the loss of intimate security in the LG is either unpleasant or threatening. Conductors have to see also the developmental opportunities LGs provide. Resistances are part of the work until participants grow more familiar and less anxious with the LG, even if already from the start many of the participants agree that the LG provides for an optimal practice space for the political and the social.

A changed facilitation of the LG towards considering it a developmental space for dialogue makes the LG fascinating and rich in variations, not necessarily having it as the exposure to its aggressive sides. Approaching the LG with the belief that it is only full of aggression rather elicits more than investigates violence. The LG dark side, by being a mass, does not need stimulation or over-interpretation to appear.

Notes

1 Temporary and affectionate name.
2 This chapter appeared previously as Friedman, R. (2016) The group sandwich model for international conflict using large groups as a social developmental space. In: S.S. Fehr (Ed) *101 Interventions in Group Psychotherapy* (pp. 83–85). New York: Routledge. The 42nd Foulkes Lecture – May 2018.

9

BEYOND REJECTION, GLORY AND THE SOLDIER'S MATRIX

The heart of my group analysis[1]

Introduction

Humans are 'social' beings. At the roots of belonging, I suggest that often rejection anxiety might be 'the' basic relational motivation. No one, no matter how socially successful, is free of rejection anxiety. And all of us have the ability to eject, split, get rid of, shake off and shut others out.[2] Clinical experience and research (Urlic, 2004)[3] show that rejection threatens the existence of group-analytic groups, while inclusion and security facilitates emotional communication. I connect inclusion with personal glory. Being 'in' provides for a glorious feeling. Inclusion in groups, communities, is experienced as success, satisfaction and health and has to be addressed in group therapy.

The clinical example that follows comes from my group-analytic group, and exemplifies a dialogue between rejection anxiety and inclusion security, trauma and glory. It has run once a week for decades: In this second session after the summer vacation seven members were present, four women and three men, aged 32 to 77, and one of them was absent. A tense participant could not wait to speak:

A (female, 42 Arabic): I want to start today, I am suffering. . . . My husband is ever more detached from me, and I am progressively drawn to a young man who works in the building next door.

B (female, 32, Jewish): I have a strong longing for a real relationship. Since my daughter was born, and even before, my husband and I have had a superficial relationship. It's difficult for us to start an intimate dialogue. He is always watching TV or busy with his phone. So hurtful . . . I am steaming with anger.

C (male, 68, Jewish): My wife doesn't seem to have any need for togetherness. She doesn't have any sexual nor any other verbal or bodily intimacy with me.

D (female, 77, Jewish): I have too much intimacy with this friend of mine. He always wants sex and always talks about the same three or four issues. The sex is great, though.

A (to D): But do you remember you said you didn't want sex, nor this man?

D: Yes . . . but I listened to the group. For the first time in my life I now have sex without guilt, without anxiety. I am devoted without restraint, I just enjoy his and my body and the relationship.

E (male, 50, Jewish): I wish I could say the same about my girlfriend. There always seems to be something I forget to do, something to feel guilty about. I really admire you – D – enjoying sex at your age.

Robi to A: When I hear the responses you got from the group, A, I wonder if you connect your husband's detachment with your attachment to someone else. Maybe his hurtful attitude is a kind of dialogue with you and your feelings for the young colleague.

A (shivering): Two days ago, I dreamt that my husband came home and saw me sitting next to the couch. On the couch lay the young man's brother. I woke up so frightened that I couldn't sleep for hours.

D: I feel now, I let myself feel the sex. I constantly think about my upbringing and education. My parents didn't let any joy, any fun or any bodily excitement into our house. They were the only two people who survived from two large families and a community. They never got over it, and I . . . and my late husband . . . he also grew up like me. I am lucky that my daughters are different. But I . . . when I caught my daughter, at the age of 22, kissing a man, it took me months to change my fear and anger about this intimacy to joy and some healthy jealousy.

Robi: to F (37, female Arab): You are silent. Can you share what's going on?

F: I am shocked that we can speak about these issues. Although I chose to come to a Jewish group so I could talk about them too, I didn't dare to do it. I love my parents, but then every time they enjoy something, they feel they are letting my grandparents down and are unfaithful to their family's misery. My grandparents had to leave their homes in their village and they never got them back as promised. And until this day I have this sadness inside me. (To D): I want to know how you got rid of this heaviness.

Robi to F:	You seem to carry all the heaviness of this group and even that of your family . . . and you seem to need someone to liberate you. . . . I want to understand it (I thought D's story and the invitation to share were 'liberations').
C: to A, the dreamer:	I want to be on your couch.
A:	(laughing) You are too old.
Robi:	(In my head: am I also too old?). It becomes important and frightening to have the choice about who is on your couch or next to it.

In retrospect I thought it was a healthy dialogue around hopes and fears, desire, glory and trauma, without 'resolution'.

(My) individual matrix

A matrix consists of the relationships and the culture of a group or society, the communication web of a community. Although we have one matrix, clinicians are used to calling the individual, the dynamic and the foundation 'matrices' instead of perspectives. What drew my attention was the matrix of exclusion and rejection, the feelings of closeness and distance. Why does 'A' panic in her dream? Is she frightened by her attraction to another man? I rather think she fears her husband's punishment and her family's potential rejection. 'D', the 77-year-old, finally feels free sexually and experiences interesting moments of glory while she is included in the group as never before. She is loved (maybe the ultimate glory) and closer to a new and free matrix. What is even more interesting: her emotional development was not facilitated by a cure of her pathological structure, but by her new matrix and its societal influences by elaborating inclusion, exclusion and rejection anxieties.

I differentiate between rejection and exclusion. Rejection is social expulsion from a group or community. It feels like death. Rejection is annihilation (Hopper). When our mother Sarah convinced our father Abraham to expel Hagar and her son Ishmael from their tents, they were rejected and condemned to die in the desert. Twice.

Exclusion is a different story. Exclusion is marginalization in the group. It connects to 'normal' Oedipal situations, where children learn to cope with marginalization and temporary non-admission to the parental presence. Exclusion is natural; it pervades our personal and professional life and is not as devastating as rejection.[4] Rejection and chronic exclusion make you sick. Inclusion cures. Rejection is trauma, inclusion is glory – extremes in a possible dialogue.

Glory has been a red rag for group analysis, with our anti-fascist history. Especially despised, and almost taboo are connections between authority and glory, like Trump's glorious promises. But, according to the Oxford dictionary, personal glory is health, happiness, contentment and social admiration, quite empowering feelings, especially its socially shared aspects. So we should rethink the contribution to therapy of a more open discourse between glory and trauma. Avoiding the use of personal glory, we may have ended up over-concentrating in therapy on trauma, while losing contact with important individual motivations, which should be named and contained. Glory can be in the same line as hope and faith, all helpful in therapeutic work. If the glory of someone is the other's trauma, then it is better to work on it, help it to find a voice, rather than only to interpret, judge or ignore! Does glory differ with gender?[5] It seems few new participants would enter our groups without phantasies of personal and social glory and secure inclusion.[6] Personally, for example, my group patients' well-being and their progressive ability to cure each other, are part of my personal glory, as are my seven grandchildren. Like many of our patients, we are greater experts on rejection and trauma than on inclusion and glory.

Here follows a personal post-emigration story of traumas and (small) glories,[7] an example of refugees, and transpersonal and transgenerational attempts to cope with rejection and trauma.

I was born into the aftermath of war. My mother escaped in 1942 from Berlin to Uruguay, South America. After the war, together with my father, who had escaped Europe earlier, they took in family members who survived the camps. The family of my childhood was preoccupied with separation, grief, survivor guilt and . . . survivor glory. They had a glorious approach to me and my cousin and loved us beyond everything. We were the jewel in the post-Shoah crown, or better . . . the piece of bread they once yearned for. Then my father died and everything collapsed again into a shortage of material and emotional nourishment, where rejections and trauma were re-enacted. For example, my mother decided to move me to the German School of Montevideo, which had just reopened, having formerly been the Nazi HQ in Uruguay. It meant that from my 5th to 13th year, I, a Jewish boy, learned in a class with 35 children of escaped Nazis, with all the consequent violence.

What made a Jewish mother, who had herself suffered from progressive exclusion and later rejection under the Nuremberg racial laws, place her son in an almost identical situation? My mother was banned from her school in Germany at the age of 13. At the same time, her friends' parents, Social Democrats who had been broken in Nazi concentration camps, then prohibited my mother from visiting their daughters after school.

Now, as a Jew in a school with the children of Nazis, my mother's exclusion was re-enacted in my class. It was not until the end of my third school year that I was finally invited by a classmate to his home. But then, when the door opened, there I was standing before 'it': a large picture of a hailing Hitler. My classmate's father, who had not been told that I was Jewish but noticed my perplexity, explained to me that Hitler was a good leader to his people. Other than in occupied Germany, in the Rio de la Plata area of Uruguay, a Nazi matrix continued to exist and live on for decades. To finish my own story about exclusion and rejection, I admit here that in spite of Hitler, I could not resist entering their home in order to play with a classmate and feel included. I think it was a good social choice, and also, after a while, I noticed that Hitler's picture was not there anymore.

I do not think my mother consciously wanted me to suffer, but exactly the other way around: she hoped that if I succeeded in surviving the ordeal, our fate as a family would change. My 'cure' by inclusion in the formerly rejecting society would also heal her own trauma. Second generations can socially cure traumas of first generations by this transpersonal 'magic'. The concept of the 'transpersonal', coined by Foulkes, implies that feelings are transported through people, and this is a cornerstone of my own thinking. Hoping the young will transform the family's fate into an 'inclusion success' is a common fantasy of transgenerational migration glory.[8] Today I believe that some wounds of rejection can only be really cured by re-inclusion by the formerly rejecting group. This includes the expelled German Jews[9] as well as the Palestinian refugees.

I hope that this story exemplifies something about the impact of social rejection, the unconscious life of hope for inclusion and glory and the use of intergenerational relations to cure trauma. I believe that members of my group-analytic group also believe that their relation to D and her new bodily/sexual relationship is curing them by contagious transpersonal inclusion.[10]

The dynamic matrix – the transpersonal in co-created group relations

Going back now to the clinical example of the group, you will remember that 'A' had a frightening dream in which her husband came home and saw her sitting next to an occupied couch.

A dream's journey starts by trying to elaborate emotional excesses with a first personal autonomous effort. Then in a second step, a dream may be told to 'partners', as a request for containment. 'A's' dreaming may be an effort to elaborate her own as well as her husband's rejection anxieties.[11] Then, by throwing her dream into the group's web, 'A' makes the second step, co-creating a shared interpersonal elaboration space. I call this two-step process dreamtelling, a combined personal and relational effort to elaborate strong emotions beyond the limited containing abilities of the dreamer herself.

Dreamtelling includes the fascinating (and weird?) possibility that 'A's' dream may also have been dreamt 'for' others. The engaged audience, the 'dreamers who dream the dream' (Grotstein, 1979), become 'A's' elaboration partners. By sharing their hunger for a warmer relationship and vulnerability to rejection, they enhance trust in the group's containment potential. In the matrix, anxiety is transformed into desire and back into anxiety. One man even wishes to replace her couch partner. For a brief moment, the group's process enacts the dream's script: a glorious phantasy of passion, and loving 'on the couch' almost ends in a nightmare. Supported by the dream, the group's dialogue between potential glory and trauma influences everyone, including me.

How is it that the interaction in a small group-analytic therapy is so open and trusting? Looking into this through the inclusion/rejection perspective, I conclude that such trust is based on what I call the 'promise' of 'no rejection' in the family. This 'promise' is an unconscious fantasy, basic to any family, even dysfunctional families, and it is transferred to the small group. Longing for the no-rejection promise seems as primary a form of social motivation as the fear of rejection. A therapy group member will seek inclusion security by the promise that no forbidden passion, no superego judgement, should result in rejecting him. Partners, co-elaborating in the dreamtelling process, by promising non-rejection, move dreams from being 'the royal road to the dreamer's psyche' to becoming 'the royal road to the mind *through* the other' (Friedman, 2002). The dream's latent communications, especially its requests for containment and demands for influence need inclusion security. This is the '*dreaming-heart*' of (my) group analysis.

The foundation matrix and the group-analytic large group

One of the Arab participants, 'F' says: 'I came to this Jewish group to talk freely about' 'Jewish' and 'Arab' societies as foundation matrices. They seem to have their own common culture and unique communication and relations. But personal growth often requires separation from one's own foundation matrix, which may be restricting thinking and behaviour. When 'F' decided to join our small group, while it seemed to be the optimal setting for working on her personal matrix, she also decided to distance herself from her foundation matrix. Actually, the optimal setting for coping with social aspects and the foundation matrix seems to be the large group. For example, in our small group, the dialogue between the Shoah and the Nakbah did not become really 'social' – it was 'only' used to share transgenerational patterns of depression and sexual inhibition. In a large group, the Shoah and the Nakbah would threaten what Volkan (2004) calls 'large group identities'. We would have substantial clashes and exchanges over territories, unacceptable guilt and power, trauma and glory. Let us now go deeper into large group processes and social phenomena.

A group-analytic approach to large groups

Over the last few decades, group analysts have progressively moved from a Tavistock style to our own approach while conducting large groups. The reason for this change is that we have taken more from our experience of conducting small analytic groups into the large group with good results. I think that there are five specific group-analytic 'positions' which have been transferred from small to large groups:

1 *The primary significance of the individual in the group.* In the Foulkesian group approach, 'the centre is the individual' (1975). Maybe we should say with Elias (1991)[12] and Mies (2017) that today: the centre is the 'group-of-individuals'. This 'individual' is not a homo clausus (Lavie, 2007; Penna, 2016), but an open, 'transpersonal' individual who should be contained in a group's context.[13]

The dialogue in the large group about personification of the individual in the 'group-as-a-whole' is just one example of such processes.

2 *Approaching groups with (increasing) trust.* 'Trusting the group', is the evolving emotional position of conductors and participants after having experienced and witnessed over the years the containment of anxieties and conflicts in ongoing analytic groups. 'A', for instance, trusted the group with a dream involving shame; 'C' trusted the group when he revealed his wishes for 'A'; and 'D' trusted the group's suggestion not to reject her boyfriend. A trusting conductor may influence the large group matrix differently than one trying to control fearful violence and psychosis (Foulkes, 1975). Becoming trustful is not utopia; it is our experience that it allows conflicts and aggression to emerge in a less anxious and stormy atmosphere.

3 *The participants' reciprocal cure.* The group-analytic group's therapeutic ability to cure is based on reciprocity between all participants, including the conductor. When 'D' says to the group: 'I listened to you', she exemplifies how dialogue (Schlapobersky, 2015) between people and feelings is the basic transformative mechanism. Group therapists learn to facilitate such reciprocal communication rather than promoting growth solely by their own unique, curative interventions.

4 *The decentralization of the (therapeutic) authority.* The conductor in group analysis has the complicated task of being an authority by providing safe boundaries on the one hand and, on the other, of developing the participants' own therapeutic authority in their own space. The conductor 'weans' the members' dependency tendencies (Foulkes, 1964: 40) by consistently moving the process from

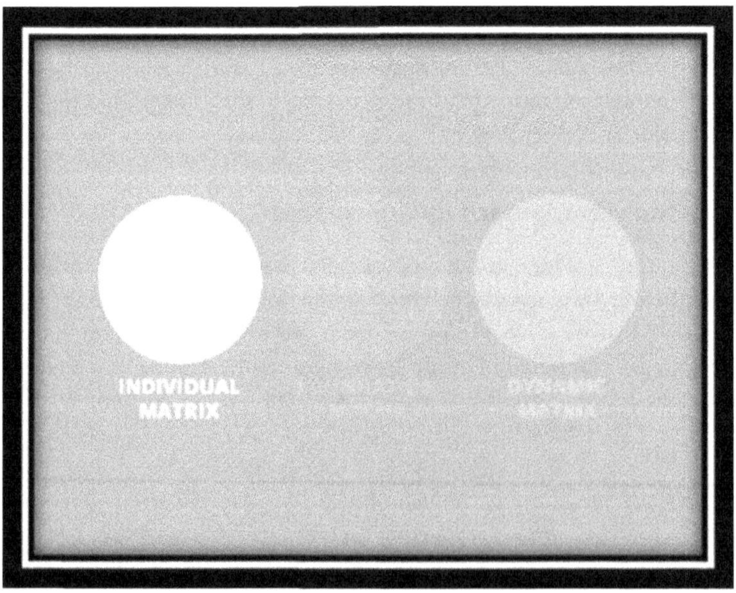

DIAGRAM 9.1 General

a leader-centred to a group-centred approach (Agazarian, 1994) which includes his own marginalization.

5 *Working with a unique 'social unconscious'.* Group analysis works with a more complex view of the 'unconscious' than that used in individual psychoanalytic therapy (Nitzgen and Hopper, 2017; Hopper and Weinberg, 2015; Mies, 2017; and Scholz, 2014). Group-analytic views unconscious processes as a tripartite matrix, or, in my words, provides a unique tri-ocular perspective on the foundation, the personal and the co-created dynamic process. In my clinical thinking, the 'individual-in-the-group', the group-of-individuals and the social context include unconscious perspectives which create a special music. They play a symphony moved by inclusion and rejection, longing and belonging, and there we often hear the sounds of trauma and glory.

A group-analytic approach to glory and rejection?

These five aspects do not only describe what group analysts seem to carry from their small group into their large group practice. They also contribute to a special dialogue between trauma and glory because they provide participants of small group-analytic groups,[14] with the longed-for promise of 'no rejection' and empower the individuals in large group-analytic groups. The non-authoritarian conduction of the 'group-of-individuals' and the facilitation of a dreamlike free communication enables a general feelings of personal and social glory, while encountering trauma.

The soldier's matrix – re-thinking societies after large groups

This concept (Friedman, 2015) promotes thinking about societies and their individuals under the influence of war threats, existential anxieties and hopes for glory. In a soldier's matrix everyone – women, children and the old – are enrolled, while soldiers are only society's delegates. All feel conscripted to identifications and efficient functioning in rather discreet and rigid 'self-less' roles. Men are called on to offer their lives in order to (gloriously) serve 'the cause'; women will again be primarily mothers of (preferably) soldiers and also serve fighters with body and soul. In my group, the traumatized parents of Jewish and Arab participants imposed a soldier's matrix with a selfless culture, excluding potential erotic feelings from their families.

A central characteristic of the soldier's matrix is that nations, subgroups and individuals progressively lose shame, guilt and empathy. Without the influence of these aggression-inhibiting feelings, dehumanization processes will not only dominate people's relation to their declared enemies but will also bring on sacrifice in general including their own children.

In the soldier's matrix leaders, rejection, traumas and glory hypnotize almost everyone, invading and occupying societies and the people's self. Everyone dreams of society's aims. I consider Israel a soldier's matrix, with all its Jewish and Palestinian citizens included.

For me, the tragedy of the soldier's matrix is that parents find glory in their children's recruitment. It repeats Isaac's Akeda/Binding (Friedman, 2017), which

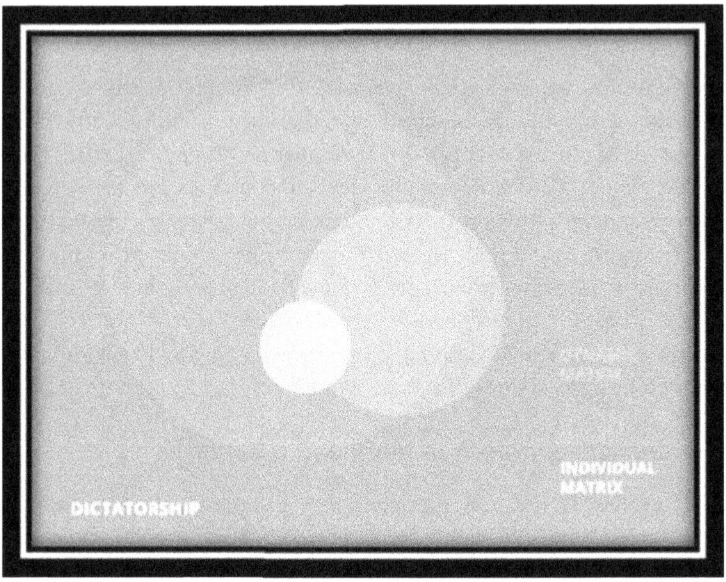

DIAGRAM 9.2 Dictatorship

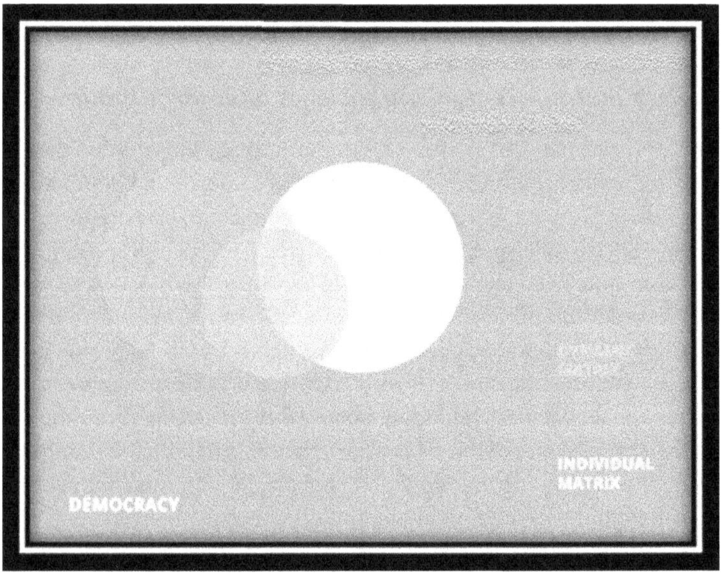

DIAGRAM 9.3 Democracy

I described in the book coedited with Yael Doron, *Group Analysis in the Land of Milk and Honey* (2017). Abraham's fear of God's rejection and his need for glorious belonging makes him pay the ultimate price: he sacrifices his beloved son. I think he over-identified with his own matrix and had a deficient selfless dialogue between his personal and his social needs. In a large group we would hope that this would be different.

Distancing from one's own matrix

I confess that finding some distance from my early total identification with my Israeli matrix took me many years. It is a long journey from being a combatant officer to be able to take up a reflective perspective. Meeting the enemy for reconciliation talks took even more time. Personal growth through a painful distancing process from one's own matrix, which a soldier's matrix often defines as 'treason', happens in groups that allow discussion of traumas and glory. The modelling of outstanding individuals, like the murdered Prime Minister, Rabin, or Amos Oz, the Israeli author, helped. 'Others', like the Germans I met at conferences 'away from the Gates of Auschwitz', who went through an inspiring distancing process from their own matrix, taught me lessons on the elaboration of rejection and annihilation anxieties.

Elias[15] described how the German soldier's matrix, incomparably the worst, came to life over centuries. Europe's possibly best educated and psycho-analysed people went into splitting processes where those who 'really' belonged were promised love, supremacy and glory, while other matrices were dehumanized and promised trauma and annihilation. It took 50 years after the Second World War ended for the children of Nazi Germany, our German colleagues, many of them sitting here,

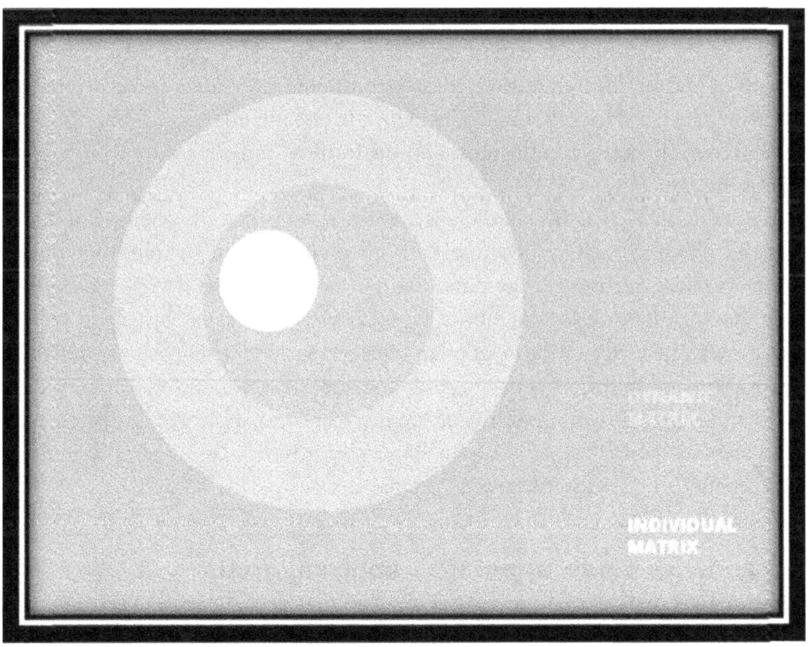

DIAGRAM 9.4 Soldier's matrix

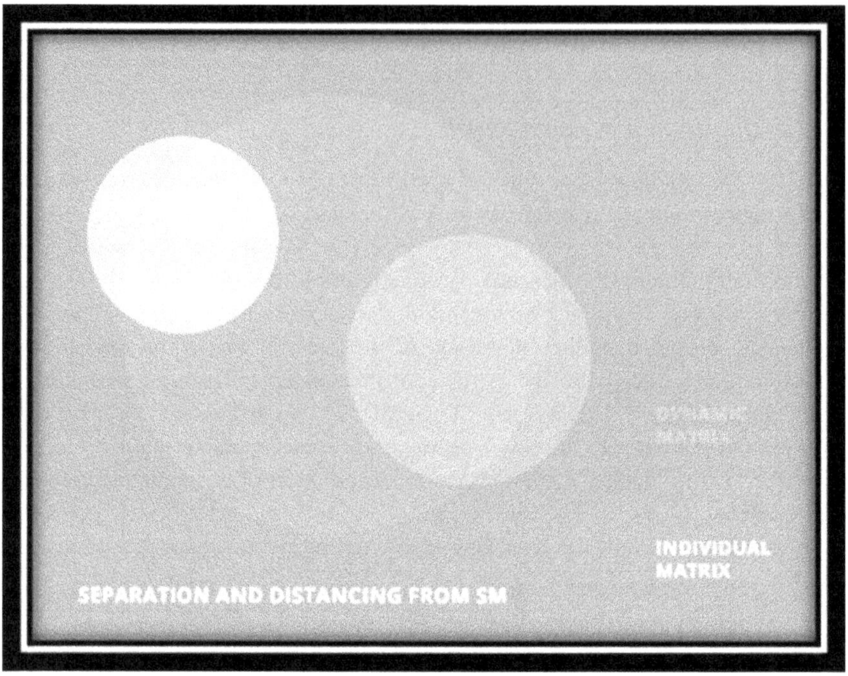

DIAGRAM 9.5 Separating and distancing from soldier's matrix

to dismantle their soldier's matrix in a difficult emotional effort. As I said at the opening of the Berlin Symposium: this is a unique, co-created and glorious social achievement assisted by other matrices. This process included painful conflicts with Germans' own parents, grandparents and institutions and a transition into an anti–soldier's matrix.

Translating this to the Israeli soldier's matrix, it seems that the opening of our civil society to pluralism, self-criticism and to our own growing awareness of the dangers of over-identification, represents a big but fragile change over the last decades. The traumas and glories of neighbouring soldier's matrices, like Syria and Lebanon, make it even more difficult to elaborate transgenerational fears, over-identification, massification and splittings between Arab and Jewish communities. I hope you may understand why it is so important for me to create and apply the sandwich model, which seems to contribute if just a small step towards the elaboration of blind social violence and inhumanity inherent in conflicts.

The sandwich model approach – applying group analysis to conflicts

Many of us who have experimented with conflict dialogue in individual and small groups learned the hard way that often these settings only provide us with illusionary reconciliation. In order to have more sustainable results in the elaboration of hate, we need to work in large groups. Why? The inclusive small group, based on the mentioned unconscious familial promise of 'non-rejection', tolerates a diversity of thinking which later is easily abandoned when in conflict with one's own matrix. The large group, on the other hand, which, similarly to society, challenges the inclusion promise, encourages a unique process in which the participants' reflective distancing stance on society's glory, hate and fear is more resilient. That's why, like Marina Mojovic and others, I find it necessary to apply large groups to civil development and reconciliation, in spite of their unfamiliar, uncanny atmosphere.

'Sandwiching' the large group between two brief small groups and repeating this setting makes it more accessible and digestible. The programme of a three-and-a-half hour evening includes a short introduction – a small group, a large group, another small group – and a short closure. For example, in Nazareth, December 2016, an Arab-Jewish organization[16] called on us when they could no longer contain emerging 'troubles'. The Nakbah, the Shoah and the Israeli Independence Day threatened to overwhelm their community with explosive emotions. Then, during the course of three evenings, 60 Jewish and 60 Arab Israelis tried to 'find their voices while listening to the voices' of former enemies. Twelve small groups were conducted by volunteers from our IIGA. Marit Milstein, Nimer Said and I co-conducted the large group.

The first Nazareth large group was rather frightening. Angry monologues of raging Arab men dominated and silenced other participants, with the exception of

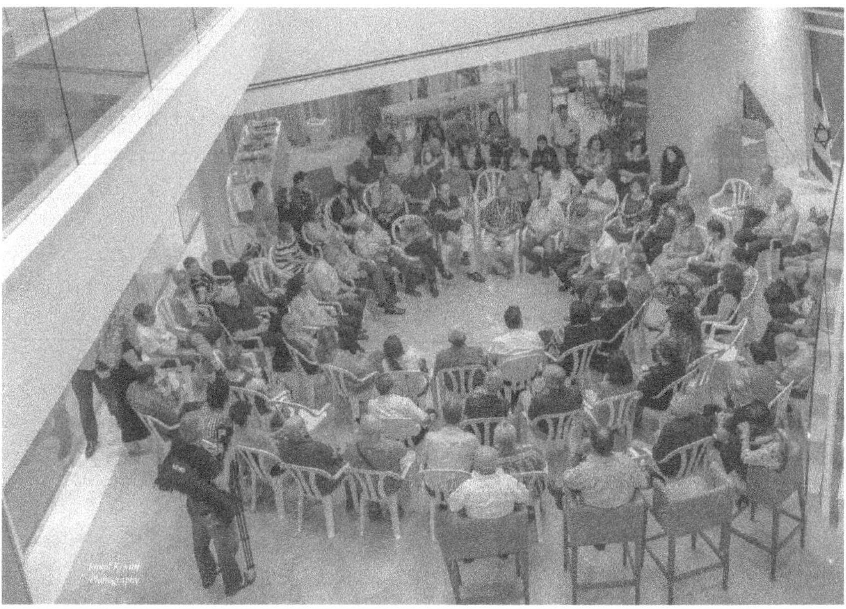

FIGURE 9.1 The large group in Nazareth, 2017

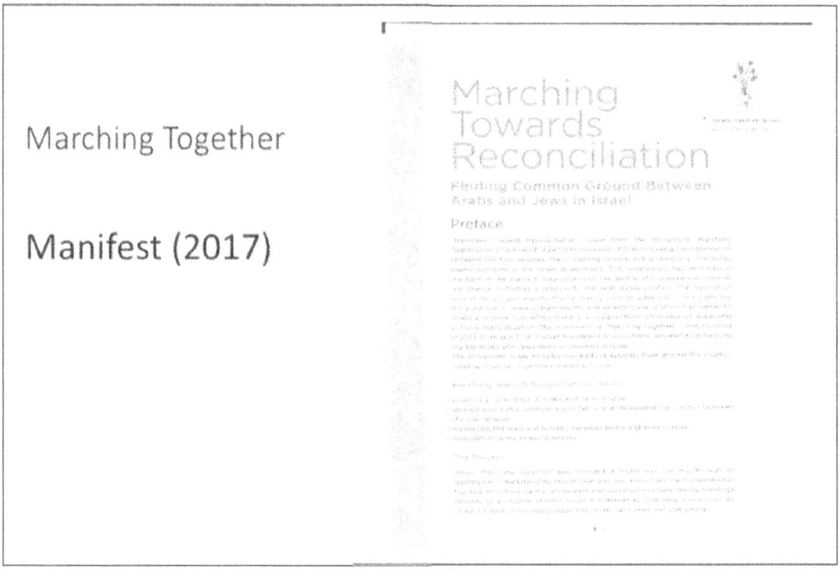

FIGURE 9.2 Manifest created by a large group as a result of the Nazareth Sandwich

a few Jewish women. I found myself acting as a traffic policeman and we barely contained the turmoil. After this first meeting we desperately needed the help of the organizers to survive the process.

Then the large group changed: the trust, which we almost lost, was regained in the second evening. Communication slowly improved and transformed the relations between the conflicting parties. Six months after the conflict-dialogue, a social treaty was written by their whole community.

I can just recommend to group analysts who are interested: try it, it is one contribution we are educated to make. This sandwich model[17] seems able to promote a difficult dialogue and understanding. It seems a journey, neither easy nor glorious.

Our experience is convincing: in this and in a split kibbutz, a village in conflict and a school, it promoted a dialogue between 'the-individuals-in-the-large-group' with conflicting emotions.

Combining small and large groups can contain the social journey in which communities grow. By having a constructive meeting, a healthier distance from our Jewish and Arab matrices was achieved. We walked together one step further away from rejection and destructive glory, in a move towards re-inclusion of Palestinians and curing the soldier's matrix. This is the social heart of (my) group analysis.

Notes

1 This chapter appeared previously as Friedman, R. (2018) Beyond rejection, glory and the Soldier's Matrix: The heart of my group analysis. *Group Analysis*. 51(4) 1–17.

2 The 'superego' and 'ego-ideal' are related intrapsychic conceptualizations of potential rejection and glory.
3 By regarding the belonging to a group as curative and suffering emotionally from rejection.
4 Only chronic marginalization, such as I described in the 'Exclusion Relation Disorder', leads to depression, anger, psychosomatic illnesses.
5 'Men kill, women love?'
6 The 'family promise', to be described later.
7 My personal story is shared to remind of the refugee history less than 80 years ago, repeated today by millions of refugees' transgenerational and transpersonal difficulties. It also pays respect to those who did their best to survive trauma.
8 Later on I also understood my mother's rejection anxiety as a 'request for containment'. But also – is this glory only a defence against trauma or a basic motivation?
9 See 'But you didn't come back' for a similar French perspective of the Holocaust.
10 As with all group-analytic concepts, rejection and glory can only be understood in relational terms.
11 Because she tells him she is afraid, ambivalent, it is in her house and she is not leaving.
12 In: Mies (2017).
13 This was Foulkes's own original position and followed by Pines and others.
14 Representing (Foulkes's fantasy of) a 'home with no-rejection' the emigrant's paradise).
15 Elias described its creation during 150 years of war ('the Germans').
16 'Marching towards reconciliation', which includes Arab and Jewish cooperating Israelis.
17 Influenced also by the human relations setting.

References

Agazarian, Y.M. (1994) The Phases of Group Development and the Systems-Centered Group. In V.L. Shermer and M. Pines (Eds.), *Ring of Fire* (pp. 36–86). London: Routledge.

Elias, N. (1939 [1991]) Die Gesellschaft der Individuen. In N. Elias (Hrsg) *Die Gesellschaft der Individuen* (pp. S.15–98). Frankfurt/M.: Suhrkamp.

Foulkes, S.H. (1964) *Therapeutic Group Analysis*. London: Karnac.

Foulkes, S.H. (1975) Problems of the Large Group. In E. Foulkes (Ed.), (1990) *Selected Papers* (pp. 259–269). London: Karnac.

Friedman, R. (2002) Dream-Telling as a Request for Containment in Group Therapy – The Royal Road Through the Other. In C. Pines, C. Neri and R. Friedman (Eds.), *Dreams in Group Psychotherapy* (pp. 46–67). London and New York: JKP.

Friedman, R. (2015) A Soldier's Matrix: A Group Analytic View of Societies in War. *Group Analysis*, 48(3): 239–257.

Friedman, R. (2017) The Group Analysis of the Akeda: The Worst and the Best Feelings in the Matrix. In R. Friedman and Y. Doron (Eds.), *Group Analysis in the Land of Milk and Honey* (pp. 61–74). London: Karnac.

Grotstein, J.S. (1979) Who Is the Dreamer Who Dreams the Dream and Who Is the Dreamer Who Understands It. *Contemporary Psychoanalysis*, 15(1): 110–169.

Hopper, E. and Weinberg, H. (Eds.). (2015) *The Social Unconscious in Persons, Groups and Societies: Volume 2: Mainly Foundation Matrices*. London: Karnac.

Lavie, J. (2007) 'Open People', 'Homo Clausus' and the '5th Basic Assumption': Bridging Concepts Between Foulkes' and Bion's Traditions. *Funzione Gammascientific Telematic Journal: Issue: Truth and Evolution in 'O' in Bion's Work*. Università 'La Sapienza' register to Tribunale Civile di Roma. www.funzionegamma.edu/inglese/number19/lavie.asp

Marching Together (2017) Nazareth: Manifesto.

Mies, T. (2017) Das kommunikative Unbewusste. Anmerkungen zum Verhältnis von Psychoanalyse und Gruppenanalyse anhand eines Fallbeispiels von Sigmund Freud bzw. Theodor Reik. Gruppenpsychother. *Gruppendynamik*, 2011(47): 151–166.

Nitzgen, D. and Hopper, E. (2017) The Concepts of the Social Unconscious and of the Matrix in the Work of S.H. Foulkes. In E. Hopper and H. Weinberg (Eds.), *The Social Unconscious in Persons, Groups and Societies: Volume 3: The Foundation Matrix Extended and Re-Configured*. London: Karnac.

Penna, C. (2016) Homo Clausus, Homo Sacer, Homines Aperti: Challenges for Group Analysis in the 21st-Century. A Response to Haim Weinberg's 40th Foulkes Lecture. *Group Analysis*, 49(4): 357–369.

Schlapobersky, J.R. (2015) *From the Couch to the Circle: The Routledge Handbook of Group-Analytic Psychotherapy*. London: Routledge.

Scholz, R. (2014) (Foundation-) Matrix Reloaded – Some Remarks on a Useful Concept and Its Pitfalls. *Group Analysis*, 47(3): 201–212.

Urlic, I. (2004) Trauma and Reparation, Mourning and Forgiveness: The Healing Potential of the Group. *Group Analysis*, 37(4): 453–471.

Volkan, V.D. (2004) *Blind Trust: Large Groups and Their Leaders in Times of Crisis and Terror*. Charlottesville, VA: Pitchstone Publishing.

INDEX

Note: Page numbers in *italics* denote references to figures.

For Product Safety Concerns and Information please contact our EU
representative GPSR@taylorandfrancis.com
Taylor & Francis Verlag GmbH, Kaufingerstraße 24, 80331 München, Germany

www.ingramcontent.com/pod-product-compliance
Lightning Source LLC
LaVergne TN
LVHW021113300926
849160LV00009B/711
* 9 7 8 1 1 3 8 3 4 6 2 8 4 *